TOUGH

TOUGH

MY JOURNEY TO TRUE POWER

TERRY CREWS

PORTFOLIO | PENGUIN

Portfolio / Penguin
An imprint of Penguin Random House LLC
penguinrandomhouse.com

Most Portfolio books are available at a discount when purchased in quantity for sales
promotions or corporate use. Special editions, which include personalized covers, excerpts,
and corporate imprints, can be created when purchased in large quantities. For more
information, please call (212) 572-2232 or e-mail specialmarkets@penguinrandomhouse
.com. Your local bookstore can also assist with discounted bulk purchases using the
Penguin Random House corporate Business-to-Business program. For assistance in
locating a participating retailer, e-mail B2B@penguinrandomhouse.com.

Photos 13 and 14 courtesy of Nana Boateng

Except as noted, all photos from the author's collection

Library of Congress Cataloging-in-Publication Data
Names: Crews, Terry, 1968– author.
Title: Tough : my journey to true power / Terry Crews.
Description: New York : Portfolio/Penguin, 2022.
Identifiers: LCCN 2021057471 (print) | LCCN 2021057472 (ebook) |
ISBN 9780593329801 (hardcover) | ISBN 9780593329818 (ebook)
Subjects: LCSH: Crews, Terry, 1968– | Men—Psychology. | Toughness
(Personality trait) | Masculinity. | Football players—United
States—Biography. | Actors—United States—Biography.
Classification: LCC HQ1090 .C7435 2022 (print) | LCC HQ1090 (ebook) |
DDC 155.3/32—dc23/eng/20211222
LC record available at https://lccn.loc.gov/2021057471
LC ebook record available at https://lccn.loc.gov/2021057472

Printed in the United States of America
1   3   5   7   9   10   8   6   4   2

BOOK DESIGN BY MEIGHAN CAVANAUGH

Some names and identifying characteristics have been changed
to protect the privacy of the individuals involved.

To my paternal great-grandfather Claude Smart
and my maternal great-great-grandfather Edward Elbert,
for leaving me such a vast and illimitable inheritance

CONTENTS

PROLOGUE

In December 2004, my wife Rebecca and I went out to celebrate. Everything in our life felt like it was finally coming together. After raising four beautiful girls, she had just found out she was pregnant with our fifth, my son Isaiah, who would be born seven months later. After I struggled for years to get by, first in the NFL and then in Hollywood, my career was finally taking off. I was hot off my breakout performances in *White Chicks* and *Friday after Next*, and Adam Sandler had cast me in his new comedy, a remake of the Burt Reynolds movie *The Longest Yard*. Since it was a football movie, and I was one of the few former pro football players working in Hollywood, it was a perfect fit. He'd even rewritten one of the characters to make sure he could get me in the film.

During the film's shoot in Santa Fe, New Mexico, I got to know Chris Rock, who was costarring. One afternoon he and I were hanging out and he started asking me a bunch of questions about being a husband and a dad. By the end of the day, he was saying, "Terry, I've got something for you. I can't tell you about it now, but I've got it. Just wait for it." That "something" was the pilot script for his new show, *Everybody Hates Chris*. He wanted me to play the father: a *lead role* in a network sitcom.

I didn't think life could get any better. The last stretch of filming on *The Longest Yard* took place back in LA, and because everything was going so well, I decided to take Rebecca out for a big celebratory dinner. We drove down to Colorado Boulevard, the big commercial strip in Pasadena, and ended up at a Spanish tapas place with live music. The restaurant wasn't even that fancy, but just being able to enjoy a night out and order steak without looking at the prices on the menu felt like a luxury compared with where we'd been only a year before. It was a perfect night, until I ruined it—and very nearly destroyed everything we had.

By the time we finished eating, it was already dark out. The sidewalks were packed with shoppers out getting ready for Christmas, and as we waited for our car at the valet parking kiosk, three black dudes came up. At the time, I wasn't really famous. Or, more accurately, I was famous only to black people. All the white folks out to dinner in Pasadena had no idea who I was. But these three dudes were like, "Hey, man! It's that nigga from *Friday*. It's Damon. Right there, man. The dude from *White Chicks*! Hey, man, lemme get an autograph and shit."

They were being loud and belligerent, and they were clearly drunk, or high. So I figured I'd make them happy and keep it moving. "Sure," I said. "You got a pen?"

Then this shit-faced dude turned to my wife—my pregnant wife—and he popped her in the arm, like a little shove. "Hey! You ain't got no pen and shit?"

"Okay, buddy," I said, pushing him back. "That's it. Back it up."

"Aw, fuck you, nigga!" he yelled. "You ain't shit! You ain't shit!"

Then he took a swing, and it was over. I saw red. I picked him up and slammed him on the concrete, and then I went at him. I stomped this dude like Nino Brown. I could feel the adrenaline surging through my body, a feeling I knew all too well from my days tackling 250-pound guys in pro football. When you get there, there's no reason, no thought process. It's pure sensation. You become hyperaware of light and sound, and you can't feel any pain and there's no stopping you. You just go.

The whole thing was a violent blur. Knowing my wife was pregnant, I was ready to kill anyone who was a threat to her. I was wearing a red sports coat, and Rebecca later said, "All I saw was this red sports coat flying around like Superman." After the one dude went down, out of the corner of my eye, I noticed the other guys looking for a cheap shot at me, so I turned my attention to them and yelled, *"Who's next?"* These two idiots looked down at their friend and then looked at each other and were like, "Uh . . . maybe not."

But the real idiot was me. Because on Saturday nights in Pasadena the cops are out. Seconds later I heard it. *Whoop-whoop!* A police car pulled over, and the officers got out. They looked nervous, itchy, hands on their guns, telling me to freeze and the whole routine. I put my hands up, trying to explain, "No, look. You don't understand. He grabbed my wife." Then Rebecca stepped in and started with the officer, saying it wasn't my fault, but this cop didn't want to hear anything we had to say. I was going to jail. He walked over, taking his cuffs out, and he was pulling my arms back behind me when this old white man walked up, waving his arms and saying, "No, no, no! I saw the whole thing, officer! This man was with his wife and this guy was bothering them. This man was protecting his wife. You've got the wrong guy."

It was literally one white guy telling another white guy, "No! You're arresting the wrong Negro! It's the other Negro!" But you know what? Thank God he did. If I'd been arrested that night, I would have gone to prison, and everything would have been over. But thanks to the word of one old white man, the cop decided to let me go. We thanked the old white guy, got our car from the valet, went on to the wrap party with Adam Sandler and Chris Rock, and played the whole thing off like a funny "Isn't this crazy?" anecdote for the rest of the night.

But it wasn't funny. It wasn't just that my rage might have ruined my whole life that night—it *had been* ruining my life, for years.

After we got home from the wrap party that night, Rebecca sat me down and said, "Terry, you have to promise me—*promise* me— that you will never ever get violent like that again. I know that man shoved my arm, but I will be okay. If you do this again, either you are going to wind up in prison or the police are going to kill you, and I'll lose you forever."

"But Becky . . ." I said.

"Nope, nope, promise me. Promise that if anything like this ever happens again, you will walk away."

So I promised her that I would. "Okay," I said. "I'll walk away."

What I didn't know at the time, what I would come to understand only with hindsight, is that I wasn't merely promising to walk away from a fight. I was promising to walk from the man I had become. I had grown up and lived my entire adult life with a false idea of what it meant to be tough. I walked around this world with my chest puffed out, like I was the alpha male. I saw myself only as strong and powerful. In fact, I was weak and powerless, and everything I did was driven by shame, insecurity, and fear.

When I promised Rebecca to walk away from that fight, I took the first step on a road to becoming a completely different person, and to become a completely different person, you need more than a promise. You need therapy. You need mentorship. You need love and support and patience from your family and friends. More than anything, you need time. As I write this, it's been seventeen years since I made that promise to Rebecca, and it's only now that I can look back and fully understand and articulate how I made the journey from there to here.

This book is the story of that journey—my journey to true power.

I

MASCULINITY

1

THE GYM

I discovered the gym when I was thirteen years old. I had never been big before. I wasn't scrawny, really, just on the skinny side of average, and being bigger had always been an obsession. I used to dream of being powerful and strong like the superheroes in my comic books.

I even had an origin story.

It happened when I was two. Toddling around the living room, I found an extension cord that was plugged into the living room wall to power a nearby lamp. I put one end of the cord in my mouth while it was still attached to the wall socket. It blew up, and I got shocked and my parents looked over to see me with a bloody, smoking lower lip with a hunk of skin hanging grotesquely from my chin. The cord at my feet told them what had happened, and they rushed me to the hospital. In the end, except for the scar I still have on my lower lip to this day, everything turned out okay, and for years I used to ask my parents to tell me the story of what happened, because to me it was like I was the Six Million Dollar Man: They had rebuilt me, made me stronger, made me into a hero with special powers and superhuman strength. When I was in kindergarten, I'd run around our house, lifting the end of the couch to see how high I could get it. One afternoon, I hoisted up the couch and felt a sharp pain in my side. I'd given myself a hernia. I was only five years old.

A week in the hospital for hernia surgery did nothing to deter me. I was obsessed with being bigger—tougher. I loved to draw, and I used to sit at the kitchen table for hours, drawing superheroes and villains with big, bulging muscles. My idol was my uncle Buddy. He had the biggest arms I'd ever seen on a man. He was a giant. Every time I saw him I'd say, "Make a muscle!" and he would. Then I'd jump on it and he'd hold me up with one arm and I would hang on to him, in awe.

Then I found the gym. Berston Field House was down the street from my school, Flint Academy, in Flint, Michigan. The gym was down in the dingy basement. It was primitive compared with what gyms are today, just pig iron, a bench, and one leg machine. But I'd do that all day, back and forth. Leg machine, bench. Leg machine, bench. At home, I would put my feet underneath my bed and do sit-ups until my stomach was so cramped and numb with pain I'd have to curl up in a ball. Then I'd wait until the feeling came back, and I would do more, going and going to the point where it would be difficult to walk.

I was obsessed with Bruce Lee, too. There was an illustrated book of exercises that was rumored to be Bruce Lee's secret, *Dynamic Strength* by Harry Wong. My brother and I would do anything to learn Bruce Lee's fitness regimen, so we ordered the book from the ads in the backs of martial arts magazines like *Black Belt* and *Inside Kung-Fu*. "Dynamic tension" is a practice of working a muscle against itself. You push your hands together, and that works your chest. You sit against a wall and hold the pose as long as you can, and that works the legs. If I couldn't be in the gym, I was doing that, to a manic degree, in the shower, in front of the TV. I'd stand there and flex my legs until the muscles cramped with pain.

This was all before Arnold Schwarzenegger and the *Pumping Iron* documentary that made him a star. This was a time when exercising every day and bodybuilding were considered strange. Everyone around me thought I was crazy. They used to look at me like, "Why are you doing all this?" I couldn't have articulated an answer at the time, but looking back now, the reason is obvious: I was getting ready to kill my father.

My father and I share the same name. Growing up I was always Little Terry, and he was always Big Terry. He was aptly named. He was a burly, intimidating man with calloused hands the size of bowling balls and a deep voice that filled me with fear. We lived in an old house with creaky floors, and when he walked, every step would reverberate through the walls—*BOOM, BOOM, BOOM*. When he stumbled home at midnight, piss drunk and spoiling for a fight with my mom, it felt like an earthquake shaking the house down to the foundation, or like Godzilla raging through downtown Tokyo, laying waste to everything in sight.

One of my earliest memories is of my dad knocking my mother out. Their fights were epic. My brother Marcelle and I shared a bedroom that was separated from the living room by only a thin dividing wall. We used to curl up in our bunk beds, petrified, pulling the covers up over our heads and listening to our father yell and stomp and bounce our mother off the walls.

The fights used to spill over into our room, too. The bedroom door would fly open and light would flood in and she would come bursting in ahead of him, telling us to get dressed, making a big show about taking us and leaving him and never coming back.

"I'm takin' the boys! I'm doin' it! I'm goin'!"

"You do that, and you'll be sorry!"

I would bolt up in bed, my heart beating wildly, scared of what was happening, scared that we might be running out in the middle of the night and, at the same time, scared that we'd be staying in the middle of this madness. But of course, we never went anywhere. It was an empty threat, a card she could play. Turning on a dime, she'd storm back out of the room, Big Terry close behind her, telling us to go back to sleep. But sleep was impossible. I could still hear them in the living room—and I'd stay up for hours waiting for the adrenaline to wear off, eventually falling into an uneasy sleep that offered no rest at all.

Eventually, as Marcelle and I grew bolder, we'd climb down out of our beds in our matching onesie pajamas and open the door a crack so we could peek through and watch the action in the other room. Mom's hair would be all messed up. Sometimes she'd be fending him off with a kitchen knife. They'd yell back and forth for what felt like forever.

"You ain't nothin'! You're a drunk. I'm sick of you."

"Leave me alone, Trish. Don't make me do somethin'! Don't make me do somethin'!"

She'd hit him and push him away and it would escalate and escalate until finally he'd haul off on her. *"You made me do this!"* POW! She'd hit the floor, and the room would go silent, leaving only the sound of her sobs.

The one saving grace was that, for all the violence Big Terry did to our mom, he never laid a finger on us. She always told him, "I'll kill you if you ever touch these kids," and he never crossed that line. But that didn't stop me from fearing that one day he might, and it did nothing to save me from the terrible feeling that consumed me every minute of every day: being powerless.

Growing up in that house, I felt like Big Terry had all the power in the world. He controlled everything—financially, emotionally, and physically. I couldn't do anything. I had control over nothing. I couldn't protect my mother, my brother, my sister. Where were the superpowers I was supposed to be able to summon at times like these? I'd ball up my tiny fists, but nothing would happen. I was too small, too weak. It's little wonder that I wet the bed until I was in eighth grade. I went to sleep terrified every night.

There were nights when I had visions of my father killing us all. He had a gun, a Smith & Wesson revolver. On New Year's Eve he'd stumble out onto the porch, drunk, and fire it in the air as soon as it hit midnight. It was terrifying. All I could do was wonder, "Is he ever going to use it on us?" Because you'd hear stories about that sort of thing all the time, especially on the local news: MAN KILLS WHOLE FAMILY. NEWS AT ELEVEN. It was always sensationalistic, to get people to tune in, which I always did. I'd sit and watch these stories about men murdering their wives and their children, and I'd think, "Yeah. My father could do that."

It was never in my mind to kill Big Terry. I never raised a hand to him; I was too scared. But I always felt a big confrontation between the two of us was coming. One day he was going to go too far, and when he did, I'd need to be strong enough to take him out. And I knew that he knew that that's what I was thinking, because he'd call me on it. "Don't you ever think you can take me," he'd say. Of course, once he said it, I couldn't help but think about it more. So I hit the gym, and I decided to make myself as big, as strong, and as tough as I could.

2

BIG TERRY

My father found his way to Flint from Edison, Georgia, one of those small southern towns with one traffic light and a set of railroad tracks separating the white side of town from the black side. I don't know a whole lot about my father's past because he never liked to talk about it. The only time he did was when he drank. He'd sit in his chair after work, obliterating himself, and all the pain and sadness would come out. "You're lucky you got a mama that loves you," he'd say, crying and slurring his words. "My mama didn't love me. My mama didn't even want me."

What I managed to piece together over the years, because it was never explained to me when he was sober, is that my dad was raised by his grandmother because his mother had abandoned him. But it wasn't like his mother was out of the picture. She still lived in this tiny town of a thousand people; he'd see her all the time. So my dad grew up in a bizarre situation. There was a woman down the street he didn't live with, but he still called her Mama. Then there was the grandmother who raised him, and she was called Other Mama. My dad had a brother and three sisters, and Other Mama raised them, too. They all had different fathers; nobody's ever told me much about any of them.

My dad left Edison at eighteen, joined the military, and after being stationed over in Germany for a while, came back to the States and followed all the other black folks heading up North to look for work. He signed on at the GM plant in Flint, eventually working his way up to be a foreman on the second shift.

My father was not without his admirable qualities. In fact, you could even say that I had two fathers. There was Big Terry before work, and there was Big Terry after work. The military had been a profound experience for my dad. It had lifted him out of poverty, given him discipline and purpose, a skill and a trade. Years after being discharged, he still dressed for work with the precision of a soldier, perfectly polished shoes and an impeccably ironed shirt with a pocket protector for his pens. As we got older, he made us iron everything we wore, even our jeans and T-shirts.

My father had an incredible work ethic, too. He was always picking up odd jobs, doing handyman work for different families around the neighborhood. He was skilled with his hands. Probably my favorite spot in the house was a wooden diner booth he'd built for us to eat in. I loved it because it made the kitchen feel like a real restaurant. "We built the pyramids, boy!" he'd say, glowing with a feeling of black pride anytime he built or fixed something. "And that's how you know we can build anything else, too."

That was Big Terry before work. After work, if we were still up by the time the second shift let off, my brother and I knew to head to our rooms the moment we heard his car pulling up outside. My father rarely drank at home. It was always out somewhere else, usually at the American Legion hall. Every now and then he'd mention the guys he drank with. It was Arthur over here or Bob over there, but I never knew my father's friends. They were like ghosts. If it wasn't the American Legion hall, he'd sit and drink and smoke in his car out in the driveway, which you could tell from the cigarette butts and Budweiser cans piled up in the back of his Chevette.

Every night it was the same routine. He'd stomp in, unsteady on his feet, and go over to the stereo console to put on his favorite record, Bobby Womack's "Woman's Gotta Have It." He'd play it as loud as he could, slumped in his chair, wallowing in self-pity. On the occasions I had to go back out through the living room later in the night, it was hard to look at him. After going to work as neat as a soldier, by midnight he'd be collapsed in a heap, his hair mussed, his T-shirt wrinkled and stained. Some nights he'd be pulled up so far inside himself he wouldn't lash out at any of us. Other nights something would set him off and the fists would come out. You never knew which way it would go.

Looking back, I know now that, in his own way, my father was fighting, and failing, to overcome his own feelings of powerlessness and fear. The ironed shirts, the polished shoes, those were his ways of asserting his worth, demanding to be treated with dignity and respect. "If you look like a clown," he'd say, "they're going to treat you like a clown. But when you look like a man, you'll get treated like a man."

But of course, that wasn't true, not for a black man in America in that day and age. As a foreman, one of the only black foremen in the whole GM shop, my father should have been in a position that accorded him status and respect. It did the opposite. The auto factories were like jail; they were run by racial cliques that all stuck together. Because my dad was so good at his job, he'd been elevated into a class of white men who never treated him as an equal. At the same time, the black workers on the floor treated him like a sellout because he was on the side of the white management. He wasn't part of either group, and he felt powerless—powerless to win over the white men who would never accept him, powerless to win back the black men who'd rejected him. More than anything, he was powerless against the alcoholism that controlled him. It was like every morning he'd wake up, put on his soldier's uniform, and head into battle. Then, every night, he'd stumble home messy and drunk, humiliated and defeated. It was the same losing battle, over and over again, every single day.

When we woke up in the morning, our dad was usually still asleep and we weren't supposed to disturb him, but of course we always did. I mostly wanted to peek in and see him because he worked a lot and I didn't get much time with him. I can remember so many mornings when I'd open the door to my parents' room, tiptoe in as quietly as I could, and watch Big Terry sleep. I'd be filled with wonder and awe. He was so strong and muscular. I wanted hands like his, big hands that seemed capable of doing anything. I'd watch him sleeping and wonder: *Is this what a man is? Is that what I'll be like when I grow up?* Then, invariably, a loud monster-like snore would erupt, and he'd roll over and I'd hurry back out of the room before I got in trouble.

I also used to sit and watch my dad getting ready for work, wanting to be close to him and learn about the ways of the world from him, but I never was able to. Sober Terry didn't like to talk. In the mornings, all I ever got out of him were clipped, one-word answers.

One morning he was polishing his shoes, and I tried to talk to him about it. "So you . . . uh, got black polish for those?" I asked, hoping to draw him out so he'd explain to me what he was doing.

"Yep," he said.

And that was it. He kept on buffing. I hung around, hoping to get more from him, but he was in a hurry and, before I knew it, he was out the door.

The only time my dad opened up—if you could even call it that—was late at night when I didn't want to be around him. He'd be in that living room chair, and he'd buttonhole me and start rambling on about grown-up things that I didn't understand, about being raised by Other Mama and not knowing his father and that whole story. Invariably he'd come around to ranting about how good my siblings and I had it. "You have it good," he'd say, again and again. I didn't understand it at the time, but it was like he was consumed with envy of his own kids. He was jealous of us for the things that he'd provided for us, and he always made it abundantly clear that, by his standards, we had nothing to complain about. We had food. We had clothes. We had a mother. We were lucky. That was especially true for Marcelle. Marcelle was my half brother, two years older than me. My mother had him when she was sixteen. Big Terry's attitude was that Marcelle should just be grateful that a new father had taken him in.

I was dying for any kind of affection or recognition from my father, and I only ever got it on a handful of occasions. Some nights he'd barge into my room, flip on the light, and stand unsteadily by our bunk bed, holding court for me and Marcelle. On one of those nights he jolted me awake and I stared at him, paralyzed as he came closer to the bed, scared of what he might do. But then he said, "Boy, I love your mother. I love you guys." I puffed up with happiness. It might have been nothing more than a sloppy, drunken confession, but it was the most acknowledgment I'd ever received. I was still smiling when he stumbled out of the room.

The next morning, Big Terry was leaning over a sheet of newspaper, shining his shoes before work as always. I strolled up to where he sat, and smiled and said, "Hey, Dad. I love you."

"Hm-hm," he said, not even looking up. It was like the night before had never happened. I was crushed. Even though I was scared of drunk, after-work dad, I started to think that that dad might be the only one I'd be able to connect with. A couple of nights later, I screwed up the courage to approach him in his chair. He was sitting there, listening to his Bobby Womack, and I leaned in and kissed him on his cheek. He turned and looked at me like I was crazy. I'll never forget it. It was a look of disgust. I backed away from him so fast I nearly tripped over my own feet.

I never made that mistake again. Whether he was sober or drunk, I kept myself apart from him as much as I could. Eventually it got to the point that if he was coming, I was going. I was scared of him. But what I was really scared of was the knowledge that, deep down, I was so similar to him.

3

ROLE MODELS

One afternoon I was chatting with Andy Samberg on the set of *Brooklyn Nine-Nine*, and he asked me, "Hey, I heard you don't drink. Is that true?"

"Yeah," I said.

"You mean you've *never* had a drink? Like, not a drop?"

"I've had a sip, but I've never liked it. Not for me."

"C'mon, you've never gotten wasted? Why not?"

"Because," I said. "I don't want to find out what would happen if I did."

And that's the truth. It's a can of worms I've never wanted to open, because I know for a fact that I would become a violent drunk like my father.

Big Terry and I were cut from the same cloth. We looked the same and had the same name, and I had his temper, too. Even as a kid, I would snap. When I was in third grade, we moved from Flint Park over to Civic Park, to our house on Winona Street. In the driveway, we had a basketball hoop where everybody loved to play because we kept the rim low enough for kids to dunk, about seven feet high. One day we were hanging out and passing around the Kool-Aid pitcher, and we started picking teams and I didn't get picked. So I lost it. I kicked everybody off the driveway. I screamed and yelled and took the ball and chucked it into the street. I remember feeling the anger rising up inside me as I was losing control, yelling, "Don't ever come back! I don't care if you ever come back!" And these were my friends. They looked over at Marcelle and said, "Man, what's wrong with your brother? We out." And they left. Even my brother took off. He was like, "I can't be around this dude." So I was left sitting there, by myself, with nobody to play with.

I had a whole summer where kids were nervous to come over. "You cool, Terry?" they'd ask before coming up the driveway. "You cool?" "Yeah, yeah," I'd say. "I'm cool." Even as a kid, I knew *I need to control my temper because I don't like being alone.* I had to behave differently so people would stay. If I didn't get picked, I would bite my tongue and say, "You guys want some Kool-Aid?" Then I'd go in the house and get some Kool-Aid and take a minute to wind down.

I don't know if my temper was something I learned from my father or if inherited it from him. It's just always been there, and I had few if any role models to show me a different way to be. My environment wasn't exactly overflowing with positive male influences. The thing that saved my life was Flint Academy, a magnet school that was the last, best hope for anybody who wanted to make it out of Flint. I loved to sketch and draw and paint, and in seventh grade, because of my talent in art, I was invited to enroll. Flint Academy was 60 percent black, 38 percent white, and 2 percent everyone else. That 38 percent white was the school's saving grace, because it meant the city still cared about it enough to not write it off the way all-black schools were, and still are, being written off all the time. I had teachers and coaches who cared about me, and all the students were encouraged to care about school and aim to go to college and make something of themselves.

As white flight gutted the city, Flint Academy was stranded like a tiny island of prosperity and hope surrounded by an ocean of crime and urban decay. There were shootings right outside the school. Gang members and drug dealers often hung around the building, waiting to put any egghead black kid or scared white kid in their place. The white kids knew to get on the bus as fast as they could to zip out to the suburbs on Linden Road, but it was open season on me and the other black kids who had to stay behind. Every day was a struggle to avoid the fate that almost certainly would have trapped me had I not been given the chance to go to that school.

During the 1980s, the Bloods and the Crips were coming up in South Central Los Angeles, and the Supreme Team was taking over in New York City. In Michigan it was no different. Down in Detroit it was Young Boys Incorporated, and in Flint we had the Top Dawgs. Young Boys Incorporated changed everything, and the Top Dawgs quickly followed suit. They soon learned that the younger you were, the better you were for the gang. You could commit a crime, go to juvie, and then come right out. So they were literally recruiting kids outside of middle schools. When I was thirteen or fourteen years old, there were kids my age getting charged with murder.

It was decimating the culture, but we didn't see that element of it at first. We saw only the cool side of it, the flashy clothes, the fine jewelry, the women, all the stuff you couldn't have because you were poor. Seventh grade is a big tipping point for most kids. It's when you finally leave toys and playgrounds behind and start looking outward, to the world of teenagers who can drive and go to the movies and hang out at the mall on their own. That's when I first really took notice of the Top Dawgs. I can remember going to the movies and seeing some fourteen-year-old kid with an Uzi in his Starter jacket and a twenty-year-old girlfriend on his arm. I was afraid of him and in awe of him at the same time, because I wanted the status and respect like he had, but I had no way of getting it.

In the first week of seventh grade, this buddy of mine, Cory, and I decided that we were going to be Top Dawgs, having no idea what that actually meant. We were going to get the jackets and the whole thing. So Cory, a naive thirteen-year-old, ran up on one of these Top Dawg guys, and he was like, "Yeah, I'm a be a Top Dawg. I'm in the gang."

This dude took one look at Cory and said, "You ain't in the gang, motherfucker!" Then he picked Cory up and slammed him on the concrete and broke his collarbone. Cory had to go to the hospital, and when he came back to school, he had a neck brace on. "Hey, man," he said, "uh, I don't think this Top Dawg thing is workin' out." That was all I needed to see. No more Top Dawgs for me. I was done.

If kids weren't drawn to gangs by the money and the status, they'd get sucked in with some pseudo-intellectual bullshit. We had all these guys hanging around my school, peddling jail knowledge. They'd go in for a couple of years, read a couple of books about the Nation of Islam or the Five Percenters, and then they'd get out and come at you with that, how "the black man is the true Asiatic king," or some other bullshit. I don't know how many times I was standing around after school only to have some dude roll up on me, going, "Listen here, young blood. Lemme tell you something. You see, the white man . . ." Then he'd go off about how being in the gang and selling drugs was about some kind of black empowerment. It all sounded hip and smart until the bodies started piling up.

Some of the boys from the neighborhood were so messed up that they started torturing animals. They'd walk around the neighborhood with slingshots, shooting at stray cats and dogs. I had a neighbor who had a pit bull on a big chain that was attached to a swing set in the backyard. He would dogfight it every night for money. We used to watch him train it. He would take the dog and make it bite down on an object hanging on a rope from the swing set. Then he'd whip it with a belt, just punish the dog like crazy to make it angry and ferocious.

I was lucky that I had a natural, healthy fear of those people. I had the good fortune to have a protector as well. His name was Chris, and he was two years older than me. His mother and my mother were best friends. We all went to church together, and I spent a lot of time over at his house. He played guitar, drums, and keyboards in the church band and was one of the most amazing musicians ever. Chris was also one of those guys who could pop a wheelie on his bike and then ride on the back wheel for two or three blocks, like a ghetto circus performer, which was the coolest thing I'd ever seen.

But if my home life was bad, Chris's was horrific. We were broke because my dad drank and gambled away his paycheck. Chris lived in abject poverty. His world was welfare and food stamps, rats and roaches crawling all over the apartment. Anytime I spent the night over at his house, I'd have to shake out my clothes to get rid of the roaches. As soon as I walked in the door at home, my mother would say, "Don't bring them roaches in my house." I had an abusive father. Chris's father was crazy. He would beat his kids with chains and extension cords and sticks that had nails in them. I saw Chris bleeding and wounded for real. I know for a time his sisters had to be taken out of the house, and I'm pretty sure it was because the dad was molesting them.

Chris used to run away all the time. We'd go over to his house to play and he wouldn't be there; he'd be gone for a week or so, getting passed through the juvie system by the cops before they'd bring him back home again. I knew he was in the streets, getting into some dirt, but he would never talk about it. The only information we got were vague warnings. "Don't go near this corner," he'd say. "Stay away from that dude."

But Chris was my protector. Because of white flight, tons of black families were flooding into these neighborhoods. There were always new people around, kids from different neighborhoods, kids from different gangs. Nobody knew each other, and because everybody had to keep up this tough-guy front all the time, there was a lot of beef. Because we'd just moved to Civic Park, we were the new kids and had to prove ourselves. From the day we showed up, there were bullies who set in on me and Marcelle and made our lives hell to let us know whose neighborhood this was.

At the time, I was at a crossroads in terms of who I was. There was the real Terry, the sensitive kid who loved art and movies and storytelling and who wanted to nerd out with my Flint Academy friends. Then there was the Terry I felt I had to be to contend with the world as I found it: my father at home and the gangs and bullies around the neighborhood. That Terry believed that he had to be as big and tough and strong and mean as anybody. That Terry also had a temper.

Even though Marcelle was older than me, I always felt it was my job to protect him. Because he'd been diagnosed with a learning disability and held back a year in school, I felt the need to take care of him. Plus I was bigger than him. If someone said something to Marcelle, I was the one to respond. One time we were walking home, and this same group of older kids started teasing Marcelle. I tried to stand up to them, but they were too big. They attacked Marcelle, beat him up, and threw him in a rosebush.

Then I told Chris about it, and I'll never forget what happened next. We showed up to school, and the kid who'd thrown Marcelle in the rosebush was sitting in the principal's office. He'd had the shit beaten out of him, and he was crying. "Why'd you get your cousin on me, man? Why'd you get your cousin on me?"

I didn't know what he was talking about. Then I went to Chris, like, "Did you . . . ?" He held up his finger to his mouth. "Shhhhh. Don't worry about it. Nobody's gonna mess with you anymore."

At the same time, Chris always told us, "But don't be like me. Don't do what I do." It was good advice. Chris ended up leaving Flint around the time I started high school. His mom got cancer and died, and he moved to Chicago. Not too long afterward, he ended up in prison. I believe it was for breaking and entering.

Part of the reason Chris looked out for us like he did was that he genuinely cared about us. I think he knew he had no way out of that life, but he was going to redeem himself for all the bad shit he did by protecting us and keeping us safe. But I think the deeper reason he did what he did was that he needed someone to look up to him. Everyone wants, and needs, respect. Everyone wants to feel looked up to by someone else. That's true of men and women, but our society makes it especially true for men. You're nothing in this world if you don't have that status. And that's what my brother and I gave to Chris. We were his audience. Anything he did, we worshipped. We made him feel like a man, and in the absence of any real male role models, Chris was the best example we had of what a man should be.

Which, when I look back, is terrifying. Chris was street smart, but that's all he was. I spent the night over at his house one time and was asking him all these questions about girls, and he started filling my head with everything he knew, most of which was wrong. "Look, man, to get a bitch, you gotta have game," he said. The "game," it turned out, was to lie. Game was making a girl believe you cared. "Tell her you love her even if you don't," Chris told me. And on and on like that. It was like learning a magic spell, playing a depressing game of make-believe, and I was nodding along, soaking it up, because he was literally the only role model I had.

The sad truth is that Chris and the Top Dawgs were boys pretending to be men. The even sadder truth is that a lot of the men in our neighborhood were men pretending to be men. I can remember going to the barbershop on Saturdays. It would take five hours to get your hair cut because older guys would walk in and cut ahead of you, and there was nothing you could do except wait. So my brother and I would sit there for hours and listen to the way these men talked. It was like a cartoon.

"I *told* that bitch she better not fuck with me. I tell all my bitches what to do."

"Man, let me tell you about these motherfuckers. These motherfuckers over here . . ."

They would rhyme and sound off like pimps, and it was all stuff they got from the movies. This was right in the post-Blaxploitation era. Everybody was doing bad impressions of Rudy Ray Moore playing Dolemite, who was a made-up caricature to begin with. If it wasn't Dolemite, it was Richard Pryor. Everyone wanted to be Richard Pryor. His cadence, his patter, they had it down.

If there was one thing that was universally true of all the men in our world growing up, it was that no matter how much they talked, they never told us anything. They never communicated with us. My father used to do this thing where he'd wake us up early, like four thirty in the morning, still dark outside. He'd knock and open the door and say, "Boys, get up." But he wouldn't explain what we were doing or what was happening. Then he'd take us to some house where we'd have to watch him fix some lady's plumbing, and we'd be there all day. But he'd never explain how long we were going to be there or why we even had to be there. He didn't *talk* to us, and it was so frustrating.

Most of my friends' dads were the same way. One of my best friends was a kid named Darwin Hall. His dad would up and leave the house and be gone for hours, and he wouldn't tell anybody where he was going. Then Darwin and I would be playing downstairs a couple of hours later and his dad would come in, look at us, say nothing, and go back upstairs, leaving us to wonder and guess what it was men do when they leave the house for hours on end every night.

There were no instructions about what being a man meant, no rituals to induct us into this grown-up world that men occupied. Anytime you learned anything it was almost by accident, an older brother who'd figured something out and maybe gave you some tips. Darwin and I got so fed up we actually made a vow to each other. We both said, "Okay, if you learn something about life before I do, promise me you'll tell me, and if I learn something about life, I promise I'll tell you." That was literally our vow. We spoke that out loud. That's how bad it was. And, of course, anytime we asked any of the men in our lives about something, they'd just chuckle and say, "Oh, you'll find out. You'll find out," leaving us to fill in the blanks. But nothing good happens when you leave young men to fill in the blanks, because when they start filling them, the bad ideas they come up with take them to all sorts of unhealthy places.

4

ANGER AND PAIN

I n its heyday, Flint was a wonderful place to grow up. My hometown was to the auto industry what Palo Alto is to the tech
industry today: an epicenter of wealth and innovation. General
Motors was the biggest corporation in the world, and it built a beautiful place for its workers to live. At school, we were always getting
on buses for trips to concerts and to visit art museums. In the summer, we'd go downtown and tons of people would be out for the big
Fourth of July parade. There was Crossroads Village, which was a
quaint old Michigan town that had been preserved as a museum,
where GM had restored a rail system from 1857 called the Huckle-
berry Railroad. It took you on a forty-minute ride along the shores
of Mott Lake and back through the little city. Even as a poor black
kid in the early 1970s, I can remember walking around my town and
thinking, "Wow, this is nice. Life is good." And it was, until it wasn't.

When court-ordered integration came to the schools, white families started leaving as fast as they could, and kept leaving for the

next twenty years. When I was in first and second grade, I lived on Flint Park Boulevard, where I still had white schoolmates and white neighbors. Ricky and Danny were the two boys in the white family a couple of houses down. My brother and I would go over to their house and play with them all the time. Then in 1976 we moved to a nicer home in mostly white Civic Park. Less than two years later, every white neighbor was gone except for old Mrs. McCauley. She worked for the phone company and was always nice. She was the only one who stayed.

Then the gas crisis hit—and kept on hitting. By the early 1980s, the auto industry was a death spiral. GM closed a bunch of its factories, unemployment soared, and the city started to crumble.

Together, the economic crisis and the racial crisis precipitated a masculinity crisis. I'd say for every ten black men I saw around the neighborhood, four of them were out of work. They had no way to support their families, no sense of purpose, no means to earn dignity and respect. They had no way to be men—at least, not according to the standards of what it meant to be a man at the time.

These guys had nothing to do to pass their days except hang around on the corner all day. All the neighborhood kids used to play football in the street, and inevitably a handful of these guys would always saunter over to get in on the action. I'm talking about grown men competing in a kids' game. Maybe they were bored or just reliving their youth, but for whatever reason they'd decided it was their job to make us tough, and they didn't mess around.

During one game, I took my position on the line, ready to get moving as soon as the play started. Then a big, grizzled man in his late twenties or early thirties, his arms roped with muscle, hunched down across from me. I was thirteen years old, and this guy was staring me down, psyching me out. "Hey, little nigger," he said. "You ain't gonna do shit in here."

The second the ball was snapped, he lunged at me. Knowing better than to show any fear, I ran at him as hard as he was coming at me. He tackled me and smacked me down on the pavement so hard I could feel the pain in every inch of my body. I lay there, gravel sticking into the back of my head, trying to catch my breath, but in an instant I was up. I knew if I showed any weakness I was done. I took hits that hard from grown men every time I played in these neighborhood pickup games. It was kill or be killed.

As I look back, it's crazy that we did that; I'd never let my son be in that situation today. One thing's for sure, though: it made me a better player. I learned to run faster and get out of the way quicker, because it hurt too much to take a hit. Whenever I did take a hit, I learned to take it without complaint. I'd brush myself off and get right back in the game. I told myself over and over: *I'm big enough. I'm tough enough. I'm fast enough. Even if they beat me today, I'm coming back tomorrow.*

My father hated football, hated sports. He believed a man should be working, learning how to build something. He always wanted me to go into the military. But when I got to Flint Academy in seventh grade, I threw myself into sports. I did it, in part, because he hated it. It was a way to get away from him, mentally and physically. Every year, I'd do football in the fall, basketball in the winter, and track in the spring. Then the next year I'd start all over again. I threw myself into every practice like it was a championship playoff game. I did extra drills on my own time. I volunteered for everything. No matter what the coaches asked us to do, I was always the first person to raise my hand.

When I hit puberty, I went through a big growth spurt. Weirdly, my hands and feet grew before the rest of my body. I was fourteen years old with size 14 feet and hands the size of Shaquille O'Neal's. When the rest of me caught up, I shot up to six foot two. I'd get to school early, hit the weight room before class, and then head straight back once my last period was out. Back then the football team had yellow-and-blue T-shirts you could earn based on what you bench-pressed. There were shirts for the 200-Pound Club, the 250-Pound Club, and the 300-Pound Club. Having one was a big status symbol at the school. When I got my 200-Pound Club T-shirt, I was so proud I literally cried. When I hit the 250-Pound Club, I'd wear that shirt until it was so dirty my mom made me put it in the laundry. I hated missing the days when it was being washed. I never made the 300-Pound Club, but there were guys who did, and I used to look at them in awe.

Being an athlete, being strong, gave me a sense of status and self-esteem I didn't get anywhere else, with the exception of my talent as an artist. In a society where people's worth is judged by their wealth, I never had much. I never had any allowance to buy nice shoes or go out to cool places. Add to that the fact that my grades were just okay. I wasn't dumb, but I wasn't an A-plus honor roll kid, so I was always scared of people thinking I was dumb. My strength and my ability on the field helped me compensate for all those feelings of inadequacy. Maybe I didn't have the prettiest girlfriend, maybe I wasn't the richest or the smartest kid in school, but I could be bigger and tougher than anybody. My body was literally the only thing over which I had some measure of control, and I used it.

It was also true that being an athlete was one of the few things that got you a pass from the gangs. You were seen as having promise. "Okay, he's got a chance of making it out. Don't fuck that up for him." Plus, if you had some neck and back on you, they'd think twice about coming after you. Still, it was hard being on the outside of that, because in the hood, gang culture defined what it meant to be a man.

Hip-hop played a big part in that. Before hip-hop, the male role models in black culture weren't tough, they were cool: Sam Cooke, Marvin Gaye, Harry Belafonte. In large part that was because black men weren't allowed to be tough. That might make the white folks nervous. Black men had to be upright and noble and nonthreatening, like Sidney Poitier and Nat King Cole. Blaxploitation and hip-hop came along as a reaction and correction to that, creating these hypermasculine figures like Shaft and Kool Moe Dee. But then it went so far that it tipped over into caricature, where you weren't a man unless you had bitches and gold chains and guns and all the rest of it. When society makes you feel worthless, you feel like the only way to counter that is to puff up your chest and assert your self-worth by being the toughest, meanest son of a bitch around. That's the essence of gang culture, which at the time was increasingly synonymous with hip-hop culture. Not all rap is like that, of course, but in the late eighties and early nineties, that was the dominant strain. Older black people heard it and were like, "What is *this*? This isn't who black people are." But in the words of Master P, my generation was all "bout it, bout it."

Still, even though that image was still the cool thing to be, I was never comfortable with it. The powerlessness and fear I felt in the face of my father was matched only by the powerlessness and fear I felt in the face of the gangs. If you stepped wrong, they would kill you, and everybody knew it. That whole thing of guys getting murdered because they accidentally stepped on some dude's Jordans was real. You could get killed for wearing a Starter jacket that a gang member wanted. You'd see them walking around wearing Starter jackets with bullet holes in them.

One afternoon I was leaving basketball practice with a new pair of Pumas my mom had bought me. They weren't anything close to the best sneakers some of the other kids had, but I loved them because they were the best that I was ever going to get. As I was walking out of practice, a guy named Julio slipped up behind me, swiped one of my Pumas from my gym bag, and ran out to the parking lot. I chased after him but stopped short as soon as I got outside. Julio was standing there, and right behind him were a bunch of the Top Dawgs, all of them sitting on the hoods of their customized Chevrolet Chevettes, with their leader, Juice, the most notorious drug dealer in Flint.

"What you gon' do, nigga?" Julio said, holding out my shoe to taunt me.

I froze. I knew if I tried to fight them, they'd kill me, but I was afraid that they'd chase me down if I ran. So I stood my ground, my heart racing.

"You better give me my shoe back!" I said, trying, and failing, to sound tough. I think I may have even stuttered trying to get it out.

Julio kept laughing. "Come get it, bitch!" he said, knowing that with his whole crew behind him that was the last thing I could do.

Finally Juice got up from his car, waved me off, and said, "Yo, give the nigga his shoe back."

Julio threw it back. It landed about five feet in front of me. I scrambled over, reached down, grabbed it, and ran.

I felt humiliated and weak, the same way I felt watching my dad beat my mom while I couldn't do anything to stop it. As with so many young men, those feelings of weakness and fear curdled inside me, turning into anger and rage. If I hadn't had football, I might have taken that rage out on myself with drinking and drugs. Without football, I might have taken it out on other kids who were younger and weaker than me. But I did have football, so I took all that rage and I poured it onto the field. Every time I got angry at my father, or at guys like Julio or Juice, I'd save it up, get in a game, and unleash. I would go all out to the point where nobody could stop me, and once I started tackling people, I felt a catharsis, a release that I'd never felt before. It's only looking back now that I understand how unhealthy it was, but at the time? It felt *good*.

People ask me about my workouts and my routine, and I always tell them I didn't get my body in the gym. I got it by hitting things at twenty-five miles an hour. We were a terrible football team, as you might expect from an academic magnet school. We'd go to tiny towns all over Michigan and just get destroyed. But I always led the team in tackles. I was never that good, if I'm being honest, but I could take tremendous amounts of pain. One of my first games, some guy hit me dead in the chest and knocked the wind out of me. I couldn't breathe. I thought my rib cage was broken. It was the most intense pain I'd ever felt. Then one of the older linebackers, a senior named Stacy, pulled me up and said, "Shake it off, man. Shake it off."

I can remember being in tears, but thinking at the same time, "I'll never quit. I have to take this. I have to endure this pain in order to make it." The strangest thing was, I felt . . . alive.

I got to the point where I welcomed the pain. "If it doesn't hurt," I thought, "you ain't doing it right." Which is a terrible thing to believe, but that was completely my mentality at the time. Pain and my ability to endure it made me feel special. I watched as other guys quit and dropped out, enjoying the feeling that I was better than them. There was one kid who took a hit, and it left him on the ground screaming. He thought he'd broken his neck. And I can remember looking at that guy and thinking, "He ain't tough enough. But I am. I can do this." I was going to show everybody.

By the time I made it to college football, I'd become a different person. My ego was out of control, and not in any way that was justified by my talents. Fully convinced that I was going to get recruited by a Division I team, I barely made it as a walk-on at Western Michigan University in Kalamazoo—with no scholarship. Freshman year, until I proved myself, I was little more than a punching bag for the older players during practice.

Still, my ego kept swelling. Part of that was, indirectly, thanks to my parents. They never let me forget how much they were paying for me to go to school. Instead of giving me a sense of humility and obligation, it had the opposite effect. I got selfish. I was going to prove to them that they were wrong for giving me such a hard time. My attitude was "If you're so resentful and stingy about supporting me, fine. I'm going make it to the NFL, and then you won't have to pay another dime for me for the rest of your life, because I'll be gone. You're making me grovel for this tuition money now, but you'll be kissing my ass down the road." And when I finally did get a scholarship, I went back home like Caesar riding into Rome. "See? I did it!" I was so pompous, so arrogant.

On the field my attitude was just as toxic. In 1988, my junior year, we won the Mid-American Conference (MAC) championship, the school's first championship in nearly thirty years, and I started making a name for myself with the scouts for the NFL. But the rage that served me so well on the defensive line was ruining everything else. I was always beefing with the other players, butting heads with the coaches. I would fight with anyone about anything at the drop of a hat.

I had made myself into a monster. Always a quiet, sensitive kid who'd been into art and comic books, after being bullied by my father and by the gangs, I'd become a caricature of masculinity. But it was all a facade. It was fake toughness I acted out because deep down I was plagued by insecurity and fear: fear that made me think I had to be the biggest, baddest motherfucker on that field, because if I wasn't, it would all fall apart and I'd be trapped back in Flint for the rest of my life.

Then, just as I barely made it into college ball, I barely made it to the pros as well. At the NFL combine in Indianapolis my senior year, I performed so well I was ranked fifth in the country for inside line-backer. My attitude was "I'm the best, and every team's going to want me." I was so cocky I left school twelve credits shy of graduat-ing with literally zero job prospects other than getting picked up by a team, even though I was flat broke with a wife and two daughters to support. I walked around telling everybody that when draft day came, I was going to go in the second round. *Maybe* the fifth.

What I didn't know, because I was young, arrogant, and stupid, was that getting drafted to the NFL is as political as anything else. It isn't only about talent. Scouts talk to coaches about players' per-sonalities and temperaments, and my coaches had been telling every team that was interested, "Hey, that Terry Crews kid. He's got an attitude. He isn't worth the trouble."

On draft day, I watched as the rounds ticked by. The phone didn't ring, and my name wasn't called. For a moment, I was actually forced to stare into the abyss. I had to wonder why it had all gone so wrong and how I had screwed it all up. Then, in the eleventh round, the Los Angeles Rams called. I'd been drafted, and they needed me on a plane the next morning.

Getting that phone call saved my life, but at the same time, it also kept me from having any kind of reckoning with myself. To me, get-ting drafted by the Rams meant everything I had done up to that point was justified. My anger and my fuck-you takeaway had gotten me everything I'd ever wanted, and my takeaway was "See? I was right." But the truth is that my anger and my fuck-you attitude had nearly cost me everything I'd ever wanted.

I've always said it takes a lot of pain to be a great football player. Guys with two loving, supportive parents are not very com-mon in the NFL. There are thousands of young men like me who fuel their athletic careers with the pain of childhood trauma or other rejections, when it should be fueled by inspiration and love of the game. But it's a recipe for disaster, because even though the pain and the anger can take you a long way on the field, once you get off it, you're still angry and you're still in pain, and you have no idea what to do about it.

5

MARLBORO MEN

For most of my youth, struggling with what it meant to be a man, the NFL player had been one of the archetypes that I and all of my friends aspired to. Carl Banks was my hero. He'd grown up around the corner from where I lived and had actually made it out of Flint to win two Super Bowls with the New York Giants. The man was a superstar to me. So when I arrived in LA for training camp with the Rams, I was walking on air. Every moment was electric. "I can't believe I'm in the locker room! I can't believe I'm in a football stadium! I can't believe this is my uniform!" I was playing on the same turf as Banks and Barry Sanders and Roger Staubach. I had joined their ranks. I was one of them, a man among men.

Except of course I wasn't a man among men. Most of the men I played with weren't men among men, either. Just like the Top Dawgs back in Flint, most of these huge, towering dudes were boys pretending to be men, hiding behind that veneer of toughness. On the field and in life, "walk it off" was the only answer to everything, no matter how traumatic. Because now, being in the NFL, unlike high school and college ball, playing football wasn't just an extracurricular activity or a means to a scholarship. Your accolades, your celebrity, your ability to support a family, your ability to pay for that ridiculous entourage to follow you around everywhere—your entire identity and sense of self-worth became wrapped up in your ability to succeed at this one thing. And in order to succeed at this one thing, you could never show weakness, never show fear, never admit to being injured or in pain. You had to carry all that inside yourself, never betraying your true feelings to anyone.

My first few days in camp, I knew I had to get noticed, and fast, or else I would fade into the sea of Rams jerseys and get thrown out. My only strategy was to fight. I took any slight, deliberate or not, as war. A shove after the whistle, even a little bit of trash talk, was a reason to start something. I was already a fairly capable actor, and even when I wasn't actually angry, I'd ham it up whenever I got into an altercation. Soon enough, I was known as a scrapper. Every time I started swinging, the head coach, John Robinson, would yell at me to cut it out. But then, as he walked away, I'd catch the faintest smirk on his face. He liked it, because it's what the NFL wants.

Half the reason I kept chasing my football dream was to get out of Flint and away from the guys like Juice and the Top Dawgs. So, needless to say, I was surprised to find out that joining the NFL meant I hadn't left the streets at all. I had teammates who were gang members. And I'm not talking about "former" gang members. These were guys with active ties to the Crips and the Bloods, and they brought all that macho bullshit into the locker room with them. The need to put up that front doesn't go away the second you get a signing bonus and a house. It takes years to unlearn. Getting those big

NFL signing checks hadn't taken these guys out of that culture. It had amplified it.

My first clue that the NFL wasn't going to be what I thought it was came during that first training camp. One of my teammates, Gerald Perry, showed up in handcuffs. I was having lunch between practices when the cops walked in the cafeteria, brought him over to the food line, uncuffed him, and let him go. I asked someone what all of this was about, and he told me that Perry had been accused of sexually assaulting his children's babysitter (which he denied). And the team let him play. The whole season. He was an offensive tackle and I was a defensive end and a linebacker, so in practice I had to go against this guy all day.

There were guys dealing drugs, and the sex was out of control. One night I got invited out with some of my teammates, and one of them pulled me aside and said, "Man, so you know, it's men only, a guy thing. No wives allowed." Not thinking too much about it, I went home and told Rebecca that I was going out with some of the players for a boys' night. She was fine with it. Then I showed up to meet the guys at a club, a place called the Glam Slam in downtown LA. They had girls crawling all over them, and that's when I realized, "Oh. They said no wives. They didn't say no women."

This was when LA was crazy. You'd go out and it was the Rams guys and the Raiders guys and the Lakers guys and the Clippers guys and rock stars and movie stars. Everybody was snorting coke in the bathroom. It was a free-for-all. This was back in the day of "she was asking for it." You'd be in the club with these guys, and the girls would come over, and the guys would put their hands wherever they wanted. If a woman ever said "No" or tried to rebuff them, you'd hear *"Bitch, what the hell?!"* and she'd get smacked.

That was the mentality, and they could get away with it because they were in the NFL. I was scared to say anything because I was new. I was barely a member of the team, and my whole identity and livelihood were wrapped up in not getting kicked off the team. I was also scared to tell my wife what was going on; it would sow mistrust in our marriage, and she'd never let me out again. So I didn't say anything. I didn't speak up and stand up for those women like I should have, as I later would when the assault actually happened to me.

It was worse on the road. Every time we arrived in a new town for a game, the first stop was a strip club. The first time we traveled to New York City, I couldn't believe I'd made it to Manhattan, the center of so much art and culture I'd always admired. The coaches told another player and me that we weren't playing the next day, so we were free to relax and play tourist. This other guy said we should hit the town together, so I thought, "Cool. I'm going get to hang out with a pro football player in New York. This is going to be amazing." It was hell. The guy grabbed a bunch of drugs and a couple of hookers, hailed a cab, and had the driver take him around in circles while he was doing his business. He only wanted me around to hang by and make sure he made it back to our hotel.

All I wanted to do was get back to my room, but I literally didn't know where we were or how to find my way around. Plus, I knew if I left him on his own and something happened, I would never hear the end of it from the team. Part of "proving you're a man" is covering for dumb shit that other men want to do. One thing I've learned is that if there's a pack of four guys, even four really good guys, something stupid is probably going to go down. Because no one wants to seem weak in front of the others. So they will do anything, *anything*, to prove that they're man enough to belong. Everything goes right over the edge, because they're all too scared to stop it.

One night the team was in Atlanta, and I didn't want to sit alone in my hotel room, so I went out with a bunch of the other players. We all met in the hotel lobby and climbed into the car of a local guy one of the players knew. The guy had a gun on him. Everybody acted like it was nothing. So, again, I didn't say anything. Fast-forward a couple of hours and, of course, being four big black dudes in a nice car, we got pulled over. One of the guys in the front seat reached back and shoved the gun at me. "Here, put this in the back!" he said. "Put it under the seat!"

I was *pissed*. This was exactly the kind of stupid shit that had made me fight so hard to get out of Flint. But I didn't have a choice at that point, so I took the gun, put it under the seat, and sat there thinking, *I'm going to jail. I'm going to jail. I'm going to jail.* All because I hadn't wanted to sit alone in my hotel room for the night.

As if the situation weren't bad enough, when the cop approached the window, the dude driving the car decided to have an attitude. "Man," he said, "why you pulling me over?" He kept on being defensive and ornery with the cop *while he had a gun in the car.* When the cop went back to his car to write up the ticket for whatever charge he was giving us, I let this dude have it. I said, "Nigga, if you give him one more word, I'm gonna hit you in the back of the head. I am not going to jail with you and your attitude."

And that was one of the tame stories. At least that night the gun didn't go off. Another time I was out in Detroit during the off-season with another player. We were walking out of a club, he and some other guys started beefing, and it escalated in the blink of an eye. It was "Fuck you, nigga!" and then *POW! POW! POW! POW!* Bullets started flying. It was the scariest sound I've ever heard. I could almost feel the air whizzing past my head. I dropped down on all fours and took off in the fastest bear crawl you've ever seen. People were screaming, car tires were screeching. I jumped in the back of my friend's car and he peeled off, almost hitting three or four people on the sidewalk. I was like, *What the hell am I doing out here?!* That was one of the scariest nights in my life. I closed my eyes and prayed, *If I ever get home, I will never talk to this dude ever again.*

I can't speak to what the NFL is like today, but the NFL I knew was like prison with money. That's exactly what it was. If you took the roster of any team I was on and you sent them to prison, in two months they'd be running the place, easy, because they're the alphas of the alphas and you've put them in a cage. Just like in prison, you can't leave. You're under contract. The team controls you. So if you have any problems with your teammates, you can't take off and get another job. You can't do the mature thing and turn the other cheek and walk away. You have to stay and you have be ready to fight. Any acknowledgment of fear or pain is viewed as a sign of weakness, and at the first sign of weakness you'll be destroyed.

Over and above all of that is the isolation. You can't trust anyone. One thing that's never talked about, but that everybody knows, is that anytime there's an injury, someone is quietly celebrating, because that's their opportunity. You're always watching your back because there's always someone waiting for you to slip. I had guys who called themselves my friends literally direct me the wrong way on the field to make me screw up a play so I'd get cut. "What are you doing covering number two?!" they'd whisper. "Go right! Go right!" So then I'd go right and the play would go sideways. Then, for everyone to hear, they'd yell, "WHAT THE HELL ARE YOU DOING, TERRY CREWS?!"

It was that manipulative, and no one there would help me, because why would they help me replace them? So nobody trusted anyone, and the coaches would play on that. It was brilliant. The coach would give a talk and then everyone would file out of the room, and the couch would say, "Jimmy, come back here. Let's talk for a second." Then everybody is left wondering, "Why did they call Jimmy?

Why didn't they call me?" You get so jealous that any camaraderie turns to hatred fast, and the NFL deliberately encouraged it.

My own position in the league was always tenuous because I was always on the bubble, always at the bottom of the roster. I walked into my first training camp with dreams of Super Bowl glory, but the truth was, I was never going to be a Carl Banks or a Barry Sanders. I was a mean, tough, athletic guy you could put out on the field to take hits, but I wasn't one of the greats. I spent seven years as a journeyman player, two years with the Rams, then a year with the Packers in Green Bay and a year in San Diego. After the Chargers cut me, I joined the World League of American Football and went to Germany to play for Rhein Fire in Düsseldorf for a year. Then it was back to the states for a year in Washington, DC, one final season with the Eagles in Philadelphia, and a miserable workout with the San Francisco 49ers that didn't even get me on the team.

It was seven years of a nomadic warrior lifestyle, and what I learned as I moved from team to team was that there were very few people I could talk to or trust. During those seven years, I played with literally hundreds of guys, and out of those hundreds of guys, I'd say five of them became true friends. Because an NFL team isn't really a "team." It's a collection of isolated and terrified men slogging through an angry, lonely existence. Everybody has to be what I call the Marlboro Man. He acts fearless, but deep down he's scared. He's in a lot of pain, but he's not telling anybody about it. Nobody likes him, and he usually dies alone.

6

THE CHRISTMAS
FROM HELL

"Your father's not doing too well," my mother said. It was 1995, my year in DC, and the auto-industry downsizing in Flint had finally come for Big Terry. His factory was closing. The layoffs were especially bad for my dad because his whole life he'd taken management's side against the laborers. He used to look at all the unemployed guys around Flint with the attitude that he was better than them, that he'd kept his job because he worked harder and was more dedicated. We'd drive down the street and see all the dudes hanging around the playground, drinking, and he would say, "These people just don't want to work, see?" Then GM sold my dad out, too.

Because he could never acknowledge what a blow it had been, my dad always called it his "early retirement." But it was a layoff. One day they told him, "Don't come back in." Then they reneged on all the commitments they'd made over the years. My dad's benefits, his pension—it all got slashed. He wound up with a fraction of what he'd been promised.

The tragedy was that, up to that point, my dad had actually been doing okay. We'd talk from time to time, and he'd voice a kind of begrudging pride about my making it to the NFL. He'd say, "Whoa. You did it, boy. You did it." Of course, he couldn't do it without taking some of the credit. "That's because I was motivating you. If you didn't have me to push against you, then it would have been too easy." Which I resented. But that's the way he was, and I took it as the best compliment I was going to get. By '95 he'd even been sober for a couple of years, too, but then GM forced him out, his depression came back, and the drinking started up again. After that, it was all downhill.

Four years later, I'd landed my first TV gig, on the reality show *Battle Dome*, and Rebecca and I finally had enough money to fly back to Flint for Christmas. I'd always promised myself that I would never let my kids be alone with my father, because I knew what he was capable of. But one night an old friend invited us down to Detroit for dinner. Rebecca wanted to go, so we decided to leave the girls with my mom and dad. I called my dad up and asked him not to drink around the girls. He promised he wouldn't, and I decided to trust him.

That night, we were driving down the highway to Detroit when Rebecca's phone rang. It was Marcelle's wife, Tramelle, and I could tell from Rebecca's face that it wasn't good news.

"Big Terry is going crazy," she said, passing me the phone. "Something is happening."

I got on the phone, and Tramelle was crying. "Big Terry hit your mother," she said. "The kids are petrified. We're taking them to Aunt Paulette's house."

So much for dinner. We pulled a U-turn and flew back to Flint. I dropped my wife off at Paulette's house and drove to my childhood home. I walked in, and it was dark, ominous, and horrible. Words can't describe how awful it was. Even the air inside the house felt different.

Big Terry had hit Trish so hard her tooth was knocked sideways, and she'd fled for Paulette's house with our kids. Big Terry was stumbling around in the little bitty kitchen, and he looked up at me as I entered.

"What the hell you want?"

"What are you doing?" I said. "What the *hell* are you doing?"

He waved me off. "Leave me alone."

"I'm grown now," I said. "And you will never lay your hands on my mother again."

Then I punched him dead in the face, and it all came back, all the times I'd cowered in the doorway while Big Terry beat my mother until she wept, all the times I'd felt small and powerless and scared. From that first punch, I flew into a rage, landing blow after blow. Today it comes back to me only in flashes; I've blocked so much of it out. I remember hitting him in his ear. All those years of pent-up anger and grief came pouring out, and I beat the shit out of him.

"Please stop," Big Terry begged. "Please stop."

"Oh, now you're gonna cry?" I said, starting to cry myself, spitting my words out through my tears. "Now you're going to ask for help? I can't believe you. Running around here having everybody afraid of you for all of those years, and now *you're* afraid?"

He took the first few punches like he was going to stand and fight, but then he started retreating, stumbling backward to the staircase, like that was going to save him, like I was going to let him get away. I beat his ass all the way across the living room to the stairs. Then I hit him in the back of the head and kicked him as he crawled his way up the stairs, yelling, "Stop! Stop!"

He managed to make it up the stairs to his bedroom, where he tried to close the door on me, and I was like, "Nah, man. No way." I pushed the door open, smacked him down to the floor, and he curled up in a ball, bloodstains on his shirt, whimpering and crying. "Don't! Don't! Stop! Stop! Please! Please!" And I kept whalin' on him. *POW!* "You deserve this!" *POW!* "Do you know how many times I had to watch you do this to her?!" *POW!* "How does it feel now!" *POW!*

I don't even know how long it went on. So much of it is a blur. At some point I couldn't do it anymore, and I fell back on the edge of his bed and burst into tears. I cried like a baby. I was filled with a profound emptiness. My whole life I'd dreamed of this moment, how cathartic it was going to feel, how *good* it was going to feel, and instead I felt nothing. It had changed nothing. It was just me beating the shit out of my own father. On Christmas. The whole thing was tragic and pathetic and sad. Even though my father had been so violent and a lot of people might say he deserved it, a real violation of nature took place that night. A son beating his father is something that shouldn't happen.

The holiday was ruined. Everybody tried to put on a happy face for the kids, but there wasn't much point. We stayed a couple of days and then flew home. I was happy to go.

I didn't set foot back in Flint for the next ten years. I put my hometown and my family in my rearview, but as the saying goes, I thought I was done with the past, but the past wasn't done with me. As a response to my abusive childhood, I'd made myself into a caricature of the big alpha male. You couldn't be "tougher" than I was. I was jacked. I was in the NFL. My first job on TV was called *Battle Dome*, a show where I was literally put in a cage to fight other men. I was still that guy, driven by a need to always be tougher, bigger, and stronger, to always be in control of everything and dominate everyone. I'd wrung a lot of success and a lot of accolades out of it, but ultimately it had brought me to a dead end. Because I didn't have any of the emotional tools or skills I needed to chart a different path, I kept running in place, repeating the same self-destructive patterns. I had no idea how to get out of it, which meant my wife and kids were stuck in it, too.

Needless to say, nothing about my time in professional football had done anything to improve my damaged sense of what it meant to be a man. If anything, it was so toxic it made me think I was perfect by comparison. I was not a good husband or a good father, but I truly believed I was a *wonderful* husband and an *amazing* father, because I'd spent my life surrounded by men who were even worse than me. There was my dad, drinking and beating his wife. There were all my colleagues in the NFL, out with different girlfriends every night. I swore I was never going to be like any of that, and to a large extent I succeeded. I said I'd never drink or abuse drugs, and I never have. I said I'd never raise a hand to my wife or my kids, and I never have. I went to college. I made it to the NFL. I settled down with a good woman and had a family. I succeeded in avoiding the worst possible outcomes for a kid in my situation, and for long time that allowed me to tell myself that I was the good guy, that I was doing everything right.

I'd tell my wife that, too. My arrogance was on overdrive. Rebecca would try to bring up problems she was having with me, and I'd be like, "What are you complaining about? You got it so good, you don't even know. Those other NFL players and how they cheat and abuse and abandon their wives? You're lucky to have me."

Rebecca was a single mom with a baby when we met, and in my mind I'd stepped in and "rescued" her with my big NFL career and Hollywood success. I look back with so much shame because I used to say that straight to her face. "You were damaged goods," I'd say. "I basically saved you. Who else was going to do that? Where would you be without me? Try and find someone who will love you more than I do." If we had a disagreement, I'd say things like "My house, my rules. You don't like it? Go. Where else are you gonna go? I got everything. I got the money. I got the whole thing. So if you feel like you've found somewhere better, go ahead."

It was a lie that I believed. The truth was, she would have done better without me, especially in those early days. She was a responsible person who actually knew how to balance a checkbook, whereas I was an immature kid with antiquated ideas that the man runs the house and the woman and the kids are just there to do what he says. Instead of having the mentality that we were a team that worked together to make a home and raise our family, I acted like I was her boss. I always had plenty to say when Rebecca did something I wasn't happy with. If she cooked a meal I didn't like, instead of appreciating the fact that she'd made a hot meal for the family, I'd pick her apart. I would actually give her a grade. My thinking was "She's a home-maker. This is her job. I get graded at work, so she has to get graded at home."

I was just as bad with the kids. Everything had to be my way or the highway. There were many, many times when, if I was mad at the kids for not doing a chore, I would walk in the house and ignore them. Which was ridiculous and immature. But my attitude was "Hey, you got it good compared to how I grew up. Ain't nobody have no mercy on me. Life is tough. Get used to it."

As the self-appointed alpha male, I was trying to control every-thing. After I started making good money on *Everybody Hates Chris*, one afternoon I took Rebecca's old car and traded it in and got her a huge black Escalade. It had rims and tinted windows and every-thing. It wasn't what she wanted at all. It was too big, too ostenta-tious, too "look at me." She'd been perfectly happy with her old car, but I ignored what she wanted because I wanted my wife to have the big status symbol. I liked how her having the car would make me look like the big shot I thought I was. I'd picked it out for her, and told her it was what she should drive, without ever asking her what she wanted. And it was the same with meals, vacations, everything. I'd always made all the decisions and expected my family to like it because it was what I wanted.

The controlled eventually becomes the controller, and after a lifetime of powerlessness, I was trying to bend the world to my will. A lot of it had to do with forcing us to be happy, even if we weren't. If the weather was gray, I wanted to turn it into sunshine. I'd adopted a mindset that was all about blinking through anything bad that happened, avoiding all negativity at any cost. This rule applied to me, and also to my family. Don't do anything that will take me down. If you're feeling bad, do something to make yourself feel good. Just get over it. After a while, Rebecca and the kids didn't want to hear it anymore. Even if they knew I was technically correct in something I was asking them to do, they wouldn't listen to me because of how I spoke to them. We would go to Disneyland, and then a big argument would start and everybody would be angry, and the whole fun afternoon would be shot. I used to ruin whole weekends with my temper. And it was all because, subconsciously, I knew my whole life was a high-wire act, a house of cards waiting to collapse. I had a pornography addiction and a hidden infidelity threatening to destroy my marriage. I was tap-dancing my way through Hollywood, a black man in a very white world, with no real idea what I was doing, afraid that it would all evaporate any minute. I was refusing to deal with years of childhood abuse and trauma that were inevitably going to catch up to me. But all I knew was to walk it off. Ignore the pain. Play through it. Move on.

What I know now is that we have to make the time to sit with the people we love and let them have their pain or their sadness. Often, that's all people need—to have their feelings validated—and they'll feel better. But at the time, I was a long way from being able to do that. It was impossible for me to sit still and feel whatever it was I was going through, and I couldn't let any of them sit and be with their feelings, either.

Looking back, I know that this stemmed from the lack of control I felt as a kid. But at the time, I didn't understand anything. All I knew was that I felt anxious and on edge all the time, even when things were going well, and the only way I knew to deal with anxiety was with rage. Always simmering underneath my out-of-control ego and my constant need for control was my anger. There were times when I would just snap. Even at the dog.

Yes, the dog.

Of all the things I've done in my life that might get me "canceled," this is probably at the top of the list, but in the interest of full disclosure, here goes. It was the summer after the Christmas from Hell, and we'd gotten a puppy named Coffee. Coffee used to eat his own shit. All the time. He would pop a squat, poop, and then turn right around and eat it. Then ten minutes later I'd see him licking my daughter's face, and I couldn't take it.

Now, up to that point I'd never done anything in my life to hurt an animal, and in my mind I never would do anything to hurt an animal. I grew up around guys in Flint who did the whole Michael Vick thing, raising pit bulls for dogfighting, just punishing them and abusing them to make them ferocious in the ring. I saw plenty of that, and it always disgusted me. But then, one day, I was out in the yard with Coffee, watching him, and he went to take a poop, and I was like, "Don't you do it!" And he did his poop and turned around and started going to town. I ran over, yelling "NO!" and I grabbed this puppy and—not knowing my own strength—I threw him across the yard. And he *flew*. He flew and he landed and he broke his leg and he yelped. At that exact moment, my daughters happened to come home. They walked in the back gate and saw everything and yelled out, "Coffee!" Then my wife came in, and everyone was staring daggers at me, like, "What did you do?"

It scared me.

"Oh my god," I thought. "I just threw the dog across the yard. What is *wrong* with me?"

I couldn't, for the life of me, figure out why I was having so many problems with my family during those years. I was successful. I was on TV. I was breaking into the movie scene. I should have been having the time of my life. But somehow we fought more than ever, and I didn't understand why.

My attitude was hurting everyone in the family, and nowhere was that more true than with my oldest daughter, Naomi. I had raised her as my own since she was two. Her biological father was out of the picture for the most part; he struggled with drug addiction, stopped paying child support, and didn't even try to contact her for many years.

Naomi was always a strong-willed child, and once she hit her teenage years, she became increasingly defiant, oppositional, and argumentative. She was an adolescent girl caught between an absent father and a difficult stepfather, acting out because she was struggling to find herself. But I was too blind to see her that way. Instead, I saw her as ungrateful and disrespectful. I was too hard and judgmental about every little thing. I would get angry if I felt she wasn't doing enough around the house or trying hard enough in school. She was a kid, but with me, she was not allowed to make mistakes. We argued constantly. There's actually a videotape of me that I'm so ashamed of. It's me yelling at Naomi as if she were a grown man, and you can see her withering beside me. After the physical abuse I witnessed and endured growing up, I told myself I was a good father simply because I never crossed that line. But a father's voice can land as hard as a punch, and mine did.

One day she finally she stood up to me and yelled, "You can't control me, Dad!"

"What are you talking about?" I said. "Nobody's trying to control you. I'm providing for you. You're living in my house."

But of course, she was right—it was about control, my obsessive need for it and my inability to attain it. One afternoon, I picked Naomi and her friends up from the mall, and they got in the car all weirded out because some skeezy dude had been leering at them and catcalling them.

These girls were fifteen years old. I asked the girls where the guy was, and Naomi pointed and said, "Over there!"

To my surprise, the guy was sitting on a bench at the bus stop. I stomped on the gas and pulled the car right where the bus was supposed to go. I jumped out and ran around the hood, and stood over him as he looked up at me.

"Yo, man!" I hollered, pointing at Naomi and her friends as they nervously watched from the back seat. "Didn't this girl tell you she was fifteen?"

"What are you talkin' about?!" he said, acting all rude.

"Didn't she tell you that she was fifteen?"

I didn't even wait for him to respond. *POW!* I straight up coldcocked this dude. He went down and hit the ground and I kept whaling on him. I looked like a pimp turning out a trick. Mind you, there were other people waiting at the stop, too. But as soon as I hit him, they split. Traffic was slowing down, and Naomi was sitting in the car, horrified in front of her friends to see her father doing this. I was so hell-bent on being "the man" protecting my family that I couldn't even see the ways in which my toxic behavior was damaging to the very people I wanted to protect. Finally, I smacked the guy one last time and got up and said, "If you see me before I see you, you'd better run, because I'm gonna kill you."

What scares me today looking back is knowing that I actually meant it, that deep down, on some level, I was fully capable of it. I spent the next week apologizing to my wife and my daughter and waiting for the cops to show up, certain that someone had taken my license plate number down. But the knock never came. If that week didn't end up with me in handcuffs, it should have at least ended up with me in a therapist's office. It didn't.

Things only deteriorated from there, and it wasn't just me. Naomi and Rebecca butted heads, too. There was one time Naomi talked back, and Rebecca snatched her by the collar and demanded she respect her parents. Naomi complained to her friends, and their parents called social services. A representative came to the house and interviewed all the kids. I was terrified that I was actually going to lose my kids that day. Luckily, we didn't. But there was no fixing things with Naomi. When she turned sixteen, she took the California High School proficiency exam, left high school early, moved out of the house and in with a friend.

I can still remember being Naomi's age, living with my father's rage and my mother's obsessive need for control, not being allowed to date or do anything I wanted, lying awake at night with a burning desire to be anywhere but at home with my family in Flint. I swore I would never be like either of them. Now, two decades later, my rage and my need for control had produced a child who hated and resented me as much as I had ever hated and resented Big Terry and Trish, which meant that somewhere I had gone horribly, horribly wrong. Two years after that, the drunk guy pushed my pregnant wife on Colorado Boulevard, and I exploded and nearly wound up in jail.

Something needed to change, but looking at yourself in the mirror and facing your demons is the hardest thing you will ever do in your life. You will duck it and avoid it—and make excuses for ducking it and avoiding it—for a long, long time. I avoided it by throwing myself into work. I threw myself into project after project, filming movies and TV shows back to back to back. I was running away from myself as fast as I could, never stopping to look down or pause for a moment's self-reflection. I did that for years, even though I knew something was deeply wrong with me, even though I'd lost my daughter and nearly put myself in jail, even though my marriage and my family were barely holding on.

Then, in February of 2010, I finally broke down and confessed my infidelity and my pornography addiction to Rebecca. We called it D-Day. It blew our marriage to smithereens, and we were left standing in the rubble, figuring out how to rebuild it—if we even wanted to rebuild it. It was a wasteland. There were days when we wouldn't speak, days when it was nothing but tears, days when everything would seem normal and then it would all fall apart. I'll be honest, every instinct in me was to run. I was afraid to sit in the mess I'd made and deal with it. There were times when I thought, "I should drive away and never come back. Everyone's hurting, and I'm the one who hurt them, so I'll just leave. I'll leave my kids. That would be the best thing for all of us. I'll wipe the slate clean and start over."

But as Rebecca and I clawed our way back, I started going to therapy and started to have small breakthroughs, epiphanies. I was so profoundly embarrassed to learn, at fortysomething years old, how ignorant I had been about the workings of my own mind—that I was so ignorant I'd been ignorant of my own ignorance. I never wanted to be in that position again, of not knowing what I didn't know, and I vowed I never would be. I developed a hunger to learn everything I could about human nature. I read everything I could put my hands on. I read books about addiction, psychology, how the brain works, anything to try to figure out what was happening with me and how I had come to end up in the circumstances I had.

It was around that time that I read a book called *Half the Sky* by Nicholas Kristof and Sheryl WuDunn. It's a book that documents the plight of women around the globe, women held in sex slavery, women subjected to rape in war—all the ways in which women are still, to this day, treated as property, as objects, by men. It hit me hard, like a blow to the chest, when I realized that that was me. For twenty years I had treated my wife as my property. Our situation wasn't nearly as brutal as those described in most of the book, of course. But it was the American version of the same story. I'd worked hard, become successful, and put my wife in a gilded cage. It had always been my mentality that I was the more important person in the relationship than her, simply because I was the man.

To this day Rebecca calls me a "recovering chauvinist." And it's true. I was a grade A, bona fide, card-carrying chauvinist. Because everything in my life, all the lessons I'd learned from my role models growing up, had told me that that was the way to be. Men were always the heroes of the story, the protagonists. Women were mere objects, trophies to be won and then controlled and, if they could not be controlled, discarded. I'd felt the same way about my daughters. Like Rebecca, they were all supporting players in the Terry Crews story, but it was always *my* story.

The deeper discovery, for me, was that my treating women and others as objects wasn't merely damaging to them. It was the thing that was destroying me. From the earliest days of my childhood, paralyzed with fear in my bed as Big Terry bounced Trish off the walls, I'd felt powerless. I couldn't change anything. I couldn't fix anything. I had no control over anything, and control was all I wanted. If I could just make my mother happy, if I could just get my father to be happy, there would be peace.

I was so desperate for that peace, I became obsessed with trying to control things I had no ability to control. But there's so much in life that's beyond your control, especially other people, particularly your wife and kids. I'd become fixated on finding the peace and happiness that I didn't have, and if I could just get my wife to do what I wanted, if I could just get my kids to behave the way I wanted, then life would be what it was supposed to be. But you can't love people and control them at the same time, because control is not love. It's manipulation. It's abuse.

The same can be true for women; any woman can be possessed by that same need to control others. What's different for men is that, from the day we are born, we're told that we *ought* to be able to control women, that we're *supposed* to control women—and if for some reason we can't control women, then somehow we've failed as men.

It's all a lie, but I had lived my life beholden to that lie, and that lie was also the thing at the root of my anger. When I look back at my life, every time I snapped and I lost it, it was always the result of something not going the way I had wanted it to, or someone not doing what I had wanted them to. When the people you think you control don't behave in the way you want, you get frustrated. When you get frustrated, you get angry. And anger, when left to fester, curdles into rage.

My father turned his rage inward with the bottle and against my mother with his fists. I thank God every day that the physical violence I inflicted in this world was never against the people I love. I poured it out on the football field and took it out on skeezy dudes hitting on my daughter at the mall—and, yes, on the dog. But words can hit as hard as fists, and I unleashed them on my family more times than I can count, and I still ask their forgiveness for that nearly every single day.

Once I had this revelation, I went to Rebecca and said, "I want to start over. I want to change." She looked at me skeptically. She started recounting all the ways I'd manipulated and controlled her and the kids, and I said, "I know." I literally got on my knees and apologized. "I'm sorry. I had it all wrong."

In the age of social media, a lot of jargon gets used and misused and overused to the point of cliché. In feminist circles, phrases like "patriarchy" and "male privilege" and "toxic masculinity" have gotten played out, almost to where you roll your eyes every time you hear them. But whatever jargon you use, the issue that's really at stake is the abuse of power.

Not all marriages are built around a male breadwinner, but our marriage was, in part because the NFL and Hollywood took us where they took us, but mostly because I'd never even allowed us to entertain any other option. In any marriage with a sole breadwinner, the breadwinner has a great deal of power. Rebecca had given me that power, and I had abused it.

Men wield power in this world because of our size and our strength, and because society gives it to us whether we deserve it or not. For almost all of my adult life I thought the purpose of having that power was to win, to dominate, to control. I felt so helpless as a kid. I had to do what everyone else said. I had to endure my father's abuse. It was always "sit down and shut up." So I made myself into the biggest, toughest man I could. But it was all a front, a fake toughness.

The purpose of being tough is not to attack, but to protect. The purpose of being strong is not to dominate, but to support. The purpose of having power is not to rule, but to serve. What I've learned is that to be a true man is to be the ultimate servant. With any talent or advantage that life has given you, whether by birth or by circumstance, your duty is to use that advantage in the service of others.

The best men I've ever known in my life, the father figures who've rescued me from having no good father of my own, have all been driven by a generosity of spirit—and not just generosity, but a creative generosity, finding new ways to share and create opportunities for the people around them, because doing so makes life better for everyone. My middle school football coach, who went out on a limb with my parents to get me on the team. My high school art teacher, who got me the scholarship that allowed me to go to college. Mentors in Hollywood like Sylvester Stallone, who believed in me and stood up for me when I didn't have the stature to stand up for myself.

In fact, I can honestly say that the toughest, most masculine thing I've ever done was not stomping a man who bumped the arm of my pregnant wife. The toughest, most masculine thing I've ever done is to come forward as a survivor of sexual assault, because it was something I did to put my strength and my power in the service of others, to try to protect the voices of those who were scared to come forward themselves.

I still have an ego—a huge, huge ego. I spent my whole life trying to satisfy that ego by getting more and more for myself: more money, more power, more control. But the ego was never satisfied, because those things can never satisfy you. But once I humbled myself and put myself in the service of others, guess what? The ego was finally sated. I was nourished. Because by using my strength on behalf of others, I was finally serving my purpose as a man.

I still have feelings of rage, too. They haven't entirely gone away. But now that I know what they are, I know how to deal with them. Anytime I'm feeling those stirrings of rage, it's coming from some feeling of insecurity, some loss of control. Somebody got a part in a movie I wanted, and now I'm worried my career is over. I had some plan or idea of how the day was supposed to go, and something's thrown it out of order. I feel that rage coming on and I tell myself, "Yo . . . relax. You're good right where you're at." Because I am good right where I'm at. Life's a game of musical chairs; sometimes you don't get a chair. You can either get mad that you don't have a chair, or choose to be happy doing something else.

I choose to be happy.

We were on a family vacation in Hawaii not long after I started to turn things around with Rebecca. My son spilled his drink at the table and it went everywhere, making a huge mess, and everyone froze. They all looked and me and held their breath, waiting for me to explode. I didn't. I grabbed a napkin and started sopping it up and I said, "Hey, man. that's okay. Everyone makes mistakes."

Rebecca and the girls could not stop looking at me, and eventually I said, "What?'

"Holy shit," Rebecca said, "you are a different person."

"What do you mean?"

"Three years ago you would have gone off if one of us had spilled that drink."

I thought back to the person I used to be, and I realized she was right. I would have lost it. I would have yelled, *"Man, come on! Do you know how much we paid for this dinner?! Watch what you're doing!"* Because I was always being driven by my own insecurities, which had nothing to do with my son having an accident.

"Terry," Rebecca said, after dinner was over and we were getting up to leave, "you're different. I can honestly say you've changed. I have never seen you that patient and that caring." Then she hugged me and said, "Now I know I've got a new man."

II

SHAME

1

WORDS AND KNIVES

Marcelle and I had heard the fighting and peeked out of the bedroom to see what was going on. Big Terry shouted at us to get back to bed, but Mom yelled, "No! Let 'em see it. I want 'em to see you hit me."

I wanted to be back in bed, but I was frozen in the doorway, standing in front of Marcelle in case I needed to protect him. Even as a kid, I knew what my mother was doing was wrong, using her kids as pawns against their father; no mother should want her kids to witness something like this. I looked over at Marcelle, and he was crying. Then I broke down and started crying, too.

"See?" my mom said to Big Terry. "See what you did to them?!"

Big Terry turned and walked out, slamming the door behind him. My mom collapsed on the floor, weeping. I took Marcelle and led the way back to our room.

My father may have been physically abusive, but my mother was no shrinking violet herself. The violence went both ways. She was no match for her husband's fists, but she could prod, taunt, and goad without mercy. She would say things to lay him low, and I learned early on that a woman can inflict terrible pain on a man by lancing his pride with a few skillfully aimed obscenities.

Words have the ability to hurt because they expose a wound that's already there. My mother would say, "You ain't nothin' but a broke-ass stinky drunk! Your mama didn't even raise you! Your mama didn't even love you!" She'd dig and dig and dig, and then *POP!* Big Terry would come back with a right hook, and it would be over.

My mother didn't have much to fight back against Big Terry besides her words and our witness, but she would occasionally deploy other weapons, like the time she stabbed him with a kitchen knife. I was five years old, and their screaming had woken me up in the middle of the night, as usual. I got out of bed and ran out and saw my father in the living room. Always the military man who was meticulous about his clothes, he had these V-neck undershirts that he wore to work. He kept them gleaming white. He was sitting there in his shirt, holding his side and yelling, "You stabbed me!" as this bright red bloodstain slowly spread across his abdomen. Then the cops came and parked their cruiser out in the driveway, lighting up the whole neighborhood with red and blue. I stood there watching it and thinking, "This is like TV. This is what you see on TV."

My mom and dad both had to talk to the cops. Then they took him to the hospital and stitched him up and that was it. In those days, nobody went to jail for that kind of thing. Nobody explained it or talked about it, either. At least not to us. The next morning it was just "Eat your breakfast and go outside and play," like nothing had happened. That time my mom actually did leave him, for a year. We went to stay outside town on a farm with her aunt, a woman we all called Mama Z. But eventually we moved back in. After that, she'd always threaten to take us and leave, but she never did.

It's never a woman's fault if she doesn't leave her abuser; the terror keeps you trapped, and I know my mother was afraid Big Terry might kill us all if she ever left for good. But there was a larger truth operating in that house as well, which was that my mother was powerless in nearly every aspect of her life. She'd had my brother when she was sixteen, followed by me two years later at eighteen. We never called her Mom. We always called her Trish. She was barely more than a kid herself, more like a big sister than a mother in many ways. There were so many times she would sit around and say, "I wish your father was dead" or "I wish he was out of here." But that's all she ever did: wish. She was powerless to *do* anything.

Most elementary school kids don't have a sophisticated grasp on human psychology, but my mother's motives were so transparent that even as a kid I understood what was happening. Her powerlessness left her with all this bottled-up anger and resentment and fear, and she had nowhere to unleash it except on the only people in her life who were weaker than she was: her children.

As abusive as Big Terry was to my mom, he never laid a finger on us; I think I got a spanking from him maybe twice, and it was nothing. But Trish would beat the snot out of us. If one of us mouthed off, *POW!*, she'd pop us right in the face. When it was bad, when I knew a real whoopin' was coming, I'd run. I ran all over that house, trying to escape her, but she always caught me. She'd make me lie down and take my pants down, and she'd get out the belt and it would be *WHAP! WHAP! WHAP!*

Screaming or crying would only make it worse. She'd be whoopin' and I'd be cryin' and she'd yell "Be quiet!" Then she'd hit me harder, which only made me scream louder, which only made her yell more. I learned to force myself to stay silent, hoping it would be over sooner if I did what she said, but the whoopings were always long and drawn out and horrible no matter what.

I lived in constant fear of her hand. My brother and sister got it bad, but I got it worse. The reason for that, I believe, is that I look like my father. I was the embodiment of her abuser, only smaller, weaker, and unable to stand up for myself. Back in the day, before everyone had video cameras, we used to make audio tapes of ourselves playing and talking. A few years ago I broke out an old cassette I had of me and my siblings playing games and singing church songs. On this tape, four-year-old me was singing a gospel song. At the time I didn't enunciate well because I had some hearing problems, so I was messing up the lyrics and *POW!*, she smacked me hard across the face. *"Stop it!"* she said. *"Sing it right!"* What's truly weird is that we used to listen back to those tapes as kids and we would laugh. "Whoa, Mom really popped you! That's hilarious!" But looking back as an adult, it's the saddest thing in the world.

When I was growing up in that house, my father's violence was so extreme that, in my eyes, he was the villain. Which meant that my mom had to be the good one, and she certainly carried herself that way. Having never learned how to stand on her own as an adult, my mother turned to one place to give structure and support to her life: the church. Only our church was not a church. It was a cult. Because Christianity is so dominant in our culture, especially in the black community, people often hesitate to refer to anything nominally "Christian" as a cult. But that's what it was. A healthy faith empowers you by giving a sense of meaning and purpose to go out and be good and do good in the world. A cult does the opposite. A cult robs you of any agency and power you might have outside the group. That's what my mother's church did to her—and, through her, to all of us.

I knew my father's actions were wrong. But because of the role religion played in our lives, I thought my mother's actions were justified, even holy. I thought I deserved all those beatings for being worthless and bad. And because I was raised in the same cult that had so deeply damaged her, I also believed I was powerless to do anything about it.

Between Big Terry and Trish, I caught it coming and going. If my father was addicted to alcohol and anger, my mother was addicted to religion and fear. Neither of them knew how to overcome, and together they made for a toxic pair. When they went at it, it was legendary. It was always brutal, and we were always in the middle.

2

TRISH

My mother used to spend days alone in her room. She'd go into a deep depression and disappear, especially after the fights with my father. Sometimes it would go a week or more. We even had a name for it. "She's in the hole," we'd say.

We moved to our house in Civic Park when I was in third grade, which was a big deal because now we had an upstairs, like the Brady Bunch, which was the coolest thing ever. There was a laundry chute, too, from the upstairs down to the basement where the laundry room was. That's where we always hung out because that's where the TV was, too. Whenever my mom went in the hole, she would shout to us through the laundry chute. It became her PA system. We'd be watching Saturday morning cartoons, and we'd hear this voice from the chute: "TERRY, TIME TO MAKE BREAKFAST!" "TERRY, TAKE CARE OF YOUR SISTER!"

We'd yell back through the chute, "OKAY!" and she'd stay in her room. At lunch and at dinnertime she'd yell for food, and we'd bring a plate up and set it by the door. Then we'd go back to watching TV and she'd stay in the hole.

It wasn't always like that, of course. Plenty of days she'd wake up sunny and bright, serving us a big breakfast without a care in the world. As a result, there was always this feeling of "I don't know who she's going to be today." Because I didn't understand why she was like that, most of the time I thought whatever was wrong was my fault.

As with Big Terry, to this day I know next to nothing of my mother's story. I know she was born and raised in Flint and that her family came from some town in Georgia, but I couldn't tell you where. Her mother, my grandmother, had been part of the migration up to Flint to work in the auto factories. She worked at AC Spark Plug for almost forty years. She sat on the assembly line, putting a nut on a bolt—the same nut on the same bolt—nine hours a day, every day, for forty years. That was considered a good job. It paid well, and she was happy to have it. She saved her money, too. My grandmother owned her house, bought the duplex next door to our house as a rental property, and even drove a Cadillac. She was set.

After World War II, my mother and her sister Paulette were born. My mom's father was a man named General Lee Simpson who was also from Georgia. Because he and my grandmother were divorced, he lived in a small house on the outskirts of town. He worked in a fish market and had a gentle toughness about him. When he smiled, wrinkles formed at the corners of his eyes, making them sparkle. He was bit of a rogue, too. He used to pick up Marcelle and me in his long, boxy Buick, a Barry White song on the radio, a toothpick in his mouth, and a straw fedora slightly askew on his head, a small feather in its band. He always had girlfriends, and we thought he was the coolest cat around.

Until my mother got pregnant out of wedlock with my older

brother, I think their lives were as comfortable as could be expected for a working-class black family of that particular place and time. I don't know too much about it, in part because we were never that close to the rest of my mother's relatives. Which was strange, because a lot of them lived nearby. We had lots of relatives in Flint, because that's how the Great Migration worked. Somebody's aunt or uncle would move up, get established, get a job, get a house. Then a cousin would come up and stay with them while they got on their feet. Then the next relative and the next and the next. So those folks from Georgia were around, different cousins and aunts and uncles. We just didn't see them.

Because we were in a cult.

My whole childhood we attended Greater Holy Temple Church of God in Christ, a Pentecostal denomination. At the center of the church was its pastor, Elder Jones, a young, handsome, and charismatic preacher. We *lived* at that church. Sunday morning services were four hours long. Then we'd go home, eat, and come right back for four more hours of the same. There was Wednesday Bible school, vacation Bible school, Friday night entertainment, everything. It was the whole hub of our lives.

The first thing a cult does is isolate you. It cuts you off from any other influences so that it can be the only voice whispering in your ear, and then it's got you. That prohibition is real, and it even extends to family. Most of my relatives were basically decent people who also had their vices. Some of them gambled. Some of them drank. Some of them listened to that devil music and went out dancing on Saturday night. Most of the men no doubt had girlfriends on the side, and a lot of them kept guns around the house, too. When you're living on the edge of poverty like we were, there's always a couple of folks around getting up to something shady. That's just how it is.

My mom would have none of it. My father had family up in Flint, too. His brother Sonny lived nearby. The few times we went over to his house, folks would be drinking and listening to music, and my mother would sit there and not talk to anybody. She had an attitude like "This is beneath me. I'm holy and I'm saved and I don't do that." She acted as if we would get dirty if we spent too much time with those people. So, of course, they didn't like her, either. They thought she was stuck up and that she was a snob, and they were correct.

Once those attitudes were established, they never really changed. We saw our relatives less and less and then eventually not at all. I'd run into my cousins at the supermarket—"Oh, hey Michelle!"—but I never had any connection to them. The only family members we stayed in regular touch with were my grandmother and her aunt, Mama Z, because they were both in the same church with my mom, and also General Lee, who was an exception because my mother helped take care of him in his old age.

Another way a cult isolates you is by cutting you off from the broader culture. Everything that I do now, movies and television and all the rest of it, is something I wasn't allowed to do then. Our church felt people were being too worldly if they listened to secular music, went to dance clubs, or went to the movies. My mother wasn't allowed to wear makeup, and the dresses she wore went all the way down to her ankles. If you wore a skirt that showed your knees, you were going to hell because you were a whore. It was damn near Amish. I wasn't even allowed to play sports until I was a teenager, and only then because the coach made a special visit to our house to assure my parents it would be a constructive, positive outlet for me.

The only indulgence allowed in that world was food, and we had more obese people at our church than the entire city of New Orleans. There was a restaurant nearby called Walli's. It had a big menu with lots of fried everything and it stayed open until one in the morning.

We would attend these late-night services, and everything would wrap up, and someone would say, "We're going to Walli's!" We'd be in there at eleven thirty at night, eating and eating and eating.

Everything we did was in the bubble of this church. If we were going to a picnic, it was going to be the church picnic. Other than events like that, we weren't allowed to go anywhere. I wanted to see and listen to what my friends were seeing and listening to, and I was lucky that I had a few people around me willing to bend the regulations. I could go to my friend Chris's house and listen to Stevie Wonder and the Gap Band. One time Big Terry broke ranks and took Marcelle and me to see *The Apple Dumpling Gang* at the theater, although he snored through the whole thing.

The big one, though, was *Star Wars*. I knew it was going to be the biggest thing ever because I'd seen the commercials for it on TV. (We were allowed to have TV, but not movies, and sometimes movies would come on TV and we were allowed to watch those, which never made any sense, but anytime I asked about it I was told not to ask any questions.) Marcelle and I didn't dare ask Trish to go see *Star Wars*, but through some miracle, our aunt Paulette leaned on my mom to let her take us to see it at the drive-in. "Trish," she said, "you *have* to let them see this movie."

Given the sheer size of the *Star Wars* phenomenon, I think my mom knew she was going to have a full-scale revolt on her hands if she said no, and after a long protest she acquiesced. Marcelle and I were ecstatic as we piled into Aunt Paulette's purple Pontiac Monte Carlo with the landau top and drove to the Miracle Twin Drive-In theater in Burton, a suburb of Flint. As the sun set, the whole parking lot buzzed with excitement. The John Williams score hit, and for the next two hours I was so enthralled I literally couldn't move. It was as thrilling as any experience I'd ever had. Immediately, I knew that making movies was what I wanted to do. It never occurred to me to be an actor, but because I was an artist, I figured I could be an animator or a special effects person. It was a life-changing experience.

Which is why the church didn't want me to have it.

My grandmother and Mama Z were both devoted to the church, but they weren't as fanatical as my mom. Mama Z would go to other churches and hear other preachers. My grandmother used to watch boxing and football and sometimes even gamble on the side. I think she drank, too, but never around us. Trish, on the other hand, took her devotion to extremes. Her zealotry grew out of her shame. She didn't like the cards that life had dealt her—pregnant at sixteen, trapped with an abusive, tyrannical husband—and she dreamed of escape. When I was a kid, she was barely in her twenties, still an attractive young woman. Men would whistle and turn their heads when she walked down the street, and in her mind, she had to be thinking about the life she *could* have had if she weren't burdened with a husband and three small children. It's why we called her Trish instead of Mom. That was at her insistence. Deep down, she didn't want to feel like a mom or accept the responsibilities of motherhood. Which shifted the parts that everyone played. We called our mother Trish. We called our grandmother Mama. And Mama Z, who was actually a great-aunt, filled the role of our grandmother.

Even though we were forbidden to go to the movies, my mother was obsessed with the world of movie stars, less for the art they created than for the glamorous lives they led. She had subscriptions to *People* and different celebrity tabloids, and she read them obsessively, cover to cover. She was addicted to Harlequin romance novels, too. Those would come every couple of weeks through another subscription she had. Whenever a new one arrived, we wouldn't see her for a few days. She'd be in up her room, reading those novels, and they kept coming and coming and coming. She probably had a thousand of them stacked up in her closet. I remember sneaking in and read-ing them once, and they were all about heaving cleavage and quiver-ing loins and quivering this and quivering that—everything was quivering.

My mother created this fantasy world in her head of this glamor-ous, romantic life she could be living, *if only*. And because those fan-tasies meant erasing her husband and children, and because church had told her living that kind of life was sinful, her fantasies filled her with guilt and shame. So Sundays brought penance, and not just penance, but catharsis.

The Church of God in Christ was the textbook definition of what people refer to as a Holy Roller church. The pastor, Elder Roger L. Jones, would start out his sermons steady and deliberate, like a train pulling out of the station. Slowly but surely, he'd ramp up into a fe-verish, singsong yell, punctuated by whooping sounds, as if he were clearing his throat, and once the preacher started "whooping," the music minister would jump on the organ, throwing in musical excla-mation points. President Camacho, the character I played in *Idioc-racy*, was based on Elder Jones. The sermons were mostly a bunch of holy words strung together, but if you listened closely they didn't actually mean anything. "When God a come down! He gonna come a down here, a heh! I give ya my word, a heh!" Everybody would be shouting along, and it wouldn't make any sense. It was more like ver-bal music, using words instead of notes, to produce an emotional response.

Once Elder Jones was rolling, people in the congregation would start to scream and jump. Then, at the climax of the sermon, the preacher would throw it to the organist, who would go to town while the congregants, overtaken by the Holy Spirit, would leap out of their pews and run around the church in a delirious haze, speaking in tongues and sometimes even frothing at the mouth. Once time a lady ran from the back of the church, down the center aisle, and slammed full force into the communion table. Then she fell to the ground and started writhing around as the "mothers" of the church— older women who were the female counterparts to deacons—draped sheets over any body parts exposed as the result of her "receiving the spirit."

All week long, the congregants were told to deny themselves any sort of earthly pleasure. And the few indulgences they did take— typically in secret—couldn't be enjoyed without drowning in feelings of shame and guilt. But then, on Sunday morning, after that week of denial and shame, they were given a release, a catharsis. Go crazy. Dance. Scream, shout, and holler. It was an endorphin rush, the only endorphin rush they were actually allowed to enjoy, and it was addictive. It was a climax, a sexual experience—and I mean that quite literally.

The Church of God in Christ was a space run entirely by and for women. Most of the husbands didn't even show up. All the "real men" would stay at home and say, "Ah, that church stuff, that's for the womenfolk. They need that." So all you had on Sundays were little boys and a handful of sexless, neutered old men in the pews. They were just there to nod and go "Mmm-hmm" to whatever their wives said.

Meanwhile, up in the pulpit was this handsome, charismatic young preacher man, and what was he doing? He was starting the ladies off slow, then building up the tempo and getting them all riled up and taking them to this explosion of ecstasy. Then they would all walk out of church going, *"Oooh!* Pastor sho' did preach to-*day!*" All that was missing was a cigarette to light up and a satin pillow to fall back on.

And that was my mother's life, this weekly cycle, a pendulum swinging from one extreme to the other. She'd lose herself in the fantasy of this romantic person she longed to be. Then, when the guilt and the shame got to be too much, she'd run back to the high-minded and moral person she felt she was supposed to be, all because she couldn't find happiness or joy with the reality of who she actually was.

Once a cult has you isolated and dependent, the next thing it does is render you powerless to control or change your own circumstances, thus cutting off any possible means of escape. In our particular religion, there was a belief that if you have faith, you can start saying what you want, and God will make it happen. You "name it and claim it"—that was the whole thing. Everyone in the church was doing this. "I'm gonna be rich," they'd say. Or "I'm gonna lose this weight." All in the belief that God was going to make it happen.

But even as a kid, I noticed that these people weren't getting what they were asking for, because they would name it and claim it, but they wouldn't *do* anything about it. It was supposed to work like magic. "Bibbidi-Bobbidi-Boo." Say the words and faith will make it happen. But then it wouldn't happen. My mom had a good friend, Dolores, who was obese. She was only in her late thirties or early forties, and she probably weighed about five hundred pounds, and she would name and claim her weight loss every day. "God, I'm going to lose this weight." But that's all she would do. She didn't change her diet, didn't exercise, and her health slowly deteriorated. By the time I went to college, she was dead. And by the logic of naming and claiming, the only conclusion you were supposed to come to was that Dolores didn't have enough faith and the devil got the best of her.

Because that was the flip side of it. Your only responsibility was to have faith. Beyond that, your problems weren't the result of your own actions. It was the devil. If you were having financial troubles, it wasn't because you were blowing your paycheck on booze every Friday, it was because "the devil was in your money." So prayer was called on to solve that, too. "I am going to bind the devil out of my finances because he has my money. I'm calling my money and all my bills paid in the name of *Jesus*!"

And that was it. That was all you, as a person, had the power to do. God and the devil have all the power, and even though God is God, the devil's got the most power. And if you have the temerity to think that you have any kind of control, that you can take responsibility for yourself and make improvements in your life, that's the greatest sin of all. Because that's pride. That's the pride of thinking you're stronger than the devil, the pride of thinking you know better than God. "Pride cometh before the fall, young man." That's what all the grown-ups would say anytime you questioned anything.

Coincidentally, around the same time, the subject of demonic possession was all over the cultural landscape. There was *The Exorcist* and the Damien movies. I wasn't allowed to see them, but all the kids would tell me about them. *Helter Skelter* had recently come out, too. The Manson murders were all anyone was talking about at school. Everyone was saying how Charles Manson could unlock the lock on his jail cell with his mind because he had the power of the devil. I thought Manson was so powerful that any day he was going to break out of prison and fly to Flint and kill me.

My problem was that I couldn't differentiate reality from fantasy because the adults in my life were telling me that this fantasy was real, that demonic possession was real, that a demon was going to take me over and turn me into this horrible, evil creature. If I had a bad attitude or I misbehaved, that was the devil making me do those things. And if that's not learned helplessness, then I don't know what is.

To make matters worse, there was an actual serial killer preying on children in Detroit at the time, a man they called the Oakland County Child Killer. He was murdering ten- and eleven-year-old boys and then bathing them and putting their clothes back on and leaving their bodies in the snow. It was always on the news. We had school assemblies about it. I was scared to death.

What really terrified me was that the only way to beat the devil was to be saved, and I never felt saved. At the Sunday services, when all the ladies in their big hats were running up and down the aisles and falling on the floor, it was because they had "received the spirit." They could *feel* it inside them, and if you couldn't feel it, you didn't have it. Elder Jones would say, "If you don't feel nothin', you don't have nothin'." And I felt nothing. I tried. I prayed for it. I begged God for it, and every week I waited for this thing that would come and take me and make me run around, shaking and speaking in tongues. But it never happened.

The even bigger fear I had growing up, above and beyond Charles Manson and demonic possession, was the Rapture. The church had a book called *Raptured,* by Ernest Angley, which described what was going to happen at Armageddon. Jesus was going to come back and take His followers up to heaven. If you weren't saved, or if you happened to be sinning at the moment He arrived, you'd be left behind on earth and the devil would be sacrificing people in the streets and his minions would cut out your tongue and cut off your head and throw it into the fire—extremely violent and brutal images. The church would give this book to kids.

Now, one of the hardest things for me to do at church was to stay awake. The services were so long and so boring and I'd get so tired, but anytime I started to nod off, I'd get the pinch—my mom grabbing my side right under my arm and pinching me awake. She used to pinch me so hard I'd practically be in tears. Then, one Sunday when I was around six or seven, I couldn't take it anymore and I fell dead asleep. There was no pinch. When I finally came to, a bit groggy and worried that Trish would be mad, I realized she wasn't there next to me. Neither were my brother and sister. I bolted upright. Everyone was gone. The whole church was empty. An intense panic came over me. It was my worst nightmare: the Rapture had come, and I'd been left behind. I'd obviously committed a sin, but I had no idea what it was.

Too petrified to move, I sat in that pew, my heart knocking in my chest. Then I heard a noise from the rear of the church. I slowly got up and crept back toward the sound. It was voices coming from the basement. Were these the other sinners who'd been left behind? Being tortured? By the time I got downstairs, I was crying and shouting, "Where's my mother? They're all gone."

From back in the crowd, my mother walked over. "No, no, no, we're here," she said. I ran to her and threw myself into her arms, relieved to discover that everyone had gone downstairs after the service to have dinner, leaving me to finish my nap. But that relief was only temporary. If anything, being "spared" that day only reinforced my conviction that the devil might get me or the Rapture might come at any moment, and that, no matter what happened, there was nothing I could do about it. I could pray to "be" saved, to "feel" the spirit. But I had no agency to actually "do" anything. I spent every waking moment powerless and ashamed and afraid.

Just like my mother.

3

DOUBLE LIVES

When I was in fourth grade, I started taking flute lessons. My mother's aunt, Mama Z, had decided that Marcelle and I should each play a musical instrument, and she'd asked us what instrument we wanted to learn. At the time, the only musician I knew was my aunt Paulette's boyfriend. They weren't married, but we called him Uncle John. Uncle John was high all the time, and he still lived with his mother. But to me he was a cool guy, a jazz man, and he played flute and saxophone. So I told Mama Z I wanted a flute. Marcelle asked for a guitar. I didn't grasp the magnitude of my mistake until the following Christmas when we woke up and underneath the tree was a guitar for Marcelle and a flute for me. The second I saw Marcelle's guitar, I knew: I should have asked for drums. But it was too late. I'd asked for a flute, so now I was a flautist.

Every Wednesday for the next four years, I had to go over to John's house after school for my flute lesson. On top of that, Trish made me practice for an hour every day. As soon as I was good enough to play in church, every Sunday I'd get up in front of the congregation in my red suit with my big black Afro and play along with the organ. I wouldn't say I was a natural-born flautist, but seeing my mother beam with pride from the pews made it all worthwhile.

Had that been the only outcome of my flute-playing career, things might have turned out okay. But flute lessons can take you to a dark place. One Wednesday afternoon, right around the time I turned nine years old, I went over to Uncle John's house for my lesson. When we finished, I went down to the basement to play and, off in the corner, not even all that hidden, came across an open chest full of pornographic magazines. Every kind you can imagine. Instantly curious, I picked up the first magazine on the top and started flipping through, gawking in disbelief at the images of naked women. I knew it was wrong, but even though it was bad—or because it was bad—I couldn't put it down. I was too young to act on it in any way. I didn't even really know what sex was, because in my ultrareligious upbringing, sex was never talked about. It was always taboo and denounced as evil, something no good person wanted any part of. Still, even if I didn't know what I was looking at, I knew I couldn't get enough of it. I liked how it made me feel, and I got a rush from doing something I wasn't supposed to do.

But I couldn't let myself look for too long. Suddenly, I got very afraid. I threw down the magazine and looked around, panicked that someone was watching. Luckily, the basement was empty; no one had seen me. But I knew God had seen me. If He'd come down to earth for the Rapture at that moment, I would have been left behind for sure. I closed the chest and ran back upstairs, promising to pray for forgiveness and swearing never to look in it again. But every Wednesday my mom made me go back for those lessons, and every

Wednesday, once my lesson was over, I couldn't help myself. The temptation was too powerful. I'd sneak back downstairs, open the chest back up, and lose myself for as long as I could.

I grew up in a world where everybody had a double life. Whenever my parents would fight, my mom would always bring it back to my dad's drinking and gambling and how he needed to get to church and get right with God. The problem was my father ran the streets, and Flint's a small town. My dad knew what was really going on with the folks at church, starting with Elder Jones. "You want me to go to *your* church?" he'd say. "Huh. That Elder Jones ain't nothin' but a—"

"Oh, don't you *talk* about Elder Jones!"

"Oh, he out there, Trish! He out there doin' all kind of stuff! You don't even know! You don't know what your people doin'."

Because what my father knew, and what my mother had chosen to ignore, was that Elder Jones was (a) sleeping with several of the married women at the church, (b) selling crack out of the pulpit, and (c) smoking a fair amount of crack himself. (All of which is true. You can read about it in his book *When Life Hurts, Dreams Fade, Hope Again*, by Bishop Roger L. Jones Sr.; he's still around preaching today.) Because my father knew this dude was crooked, whenever my mom threw religion in his face, he would go off on her. He would never come out and tell her the whole truth, because he knew the church was all she had, and he didn't want to ruin it for her. At the same time, he didn't want to listen to her sermons.

Of course, Elder Jones wasn't the only one at church leading a double life. Homosexuality was loudly denounced, but the choir director was gay. He had boyfriends on the side. Everybody knew, but it was always "don't ask, don't tell." As long as he stayed in the closet to give everyone plausible deniability, nothing was ever said.

At least forcing the choir director to hide his personal life didn't harm anyone except the choir director. The church's sexual hypocrisy had other, darker consequences as well. There were child molesters in the congregation, serial abusers. The older kids would warn you about them.

"Yo, don't go anywhere with that dude. Don't get in his car."

"Why not?"

"He'll turn you out."

My mother knew who they were, too, and she'd quietly steer me and Marcelle away from them. But she'd never actually say anything, and these guys would go on hunting for other victims.

All of that was going on right underneath the surface, men cheating on their wives, women getting pregnant by men who weren't their husbands. There were fathers you looked up to as good and decent and holy, and then one day you'd find out they had a whole other family living across town. And of course there was my mother, holing up with her romance novels all week and then walking out the door every Sunday morning being all holier than thou.

People had plenty of secrets they liked to keep hidden outside the church, too. My father had other women. They would call the house, which would cause Big Terry and Trish to have another huge blowout, only to go right back to pretending nothing had happened. My mom's younger sister Marquita was only a few years older than us, and she got hit by the crack epidemic hard. She would steal anything she could get her hands on. She even stole my grandmother's riding lawn mower in the middle of a snowstorm; there were tracks in the snow from the garage out to the street where she took off in the middle of a blizzard to go sell the thing for crack. But again, none of it was ever explained or talked about.

Which is not uncommon. Everybody keeps secrets. But our church was so strict and so oppressive that people took things to extremes. People would put a TV on the windowsill and watch the TV on the windowsill and then go to church and say, "I don't have a TV in my house." That's the level of dissonance that we're talking about.

It was all about the image you projected and not about who you actually were. When I was growing up, the message to me was clear: You show one face to the world, and that face is always upright and virtuous. Anything that's dark and sinful and weak, you hide it away and don't talk about it. If you're out there openly drinking and gambling and fornicating, you'll be publicly denounced and shamed and excommunicated. But as long as you maintain the virtuous facade and keep the darkness hidden away, nobody will ever say anything.

Which brings me back to the chest of magazines in Uncle John's basement. What I found down there wasn't really about sex, or not entirely about sex. What I found was numbness. Porn gave me an escape. I would unplug from my life and forget about all the violence and the fighting and the drinking and the church and the anxiety and the pressure. I lived in fear of my parents, in fear of the devil, and the only time I wasn't scared was when I was looking at porn, because it sucked me in and the rest of the world just fell away.

Of course, as soon as I put the porn down, I'd be gripped by an even greater fear: that I would get caught. Either by my parents, which would be bad. Or by the devil, because it would be just my luck that the Rapture would come while I was down in Uncle John's basement looking at *Penthouse*. The trips to the basement were always followed by some bout of intense anxiety, so every week I'd head home from my lessons filled with even more shame and fear. I'd pray all night long. "I'll never do it again. I'll never do it again. I'll never do it again." I'd lie awake, filled with so much fear, and the only thing that could make the fear go away was more porn. So every time I went over to my aunt's house, I'd go right back down to the basement to numb myself again.

Pretty soon, the chest in Uncle John's basement wouldn't suffice.

I was looking for porn anywhere I could find it. Which wasn't too difficult. Back then drugstores still carried adult magazines. There would be copies of *Playboy* and *Oui* and *Hustler* right next to *People* magazine. While Trish was running her errands, I'd tell her I was going to the drugstore to look at comic books, and then I'd duck into the magazine aisle and flip through the images for as long as I could get away with.

More than once my reverie was interrupted by a familiar scolding voice as Trish came running up the aisle.

"Boy!" she'd say. "What are you looking at?"

I'd quickly toss the magazine back on the shelf and pretend to have no idea what she was talking about. Then she'd pretend she hadn't seen me, either. Because in order to discipline me, she'd have to acknowledge what I'd been exposed to, and she wasn't about to sit down and have a real conversation with me about sex or anything else.

You'd think, given that my mother had gotten pregnant as a teenager, she might have instructed us on how not to let that happen. But there was no birds and the bees talk in our house, so on top of all the unhealthy reasons I was so drawn to porn, one was simple curiosity. Nobody ever told me what sex was or what it was for or how any of it worked. Porn was my only education, and it wasn't a good one. But because my mother couldn't acknowledge anything unsavory, like my father's affairs or my aunt's crack habit, my burgeoning fascination with porn was one more thing for her to be in denial about.

It wasn't long before I graduated to video. My friend JoNathan from church had learned how to rig his family's cable box so that the adult channel, Escapade, came through. We started watching it every chance we got. It was the first time I'd seen pornographic movies, which were way better than the magazines. Not only were they full of sex, but a lot of them were warped versions of children's stories: *Jack and Jill* and *Alice in Wonderland* and *Goldilocks*. It didn't take me long to figure out how to rig our cable box the same way.

Once I had access to pornography in the house, it really became a problem. I watched it every chance I got. Marcelle watched it, too. But then one day he came into the living room, caught sight of the TV, and stopped short.

"Man, I'm not doing that anymore," he said. "I don't need it."

I stared at him for a long time. "Shoot, you go ahead," I said. "I'm gonna watch."

I felt guilty as he went upstairs without me, but I couldn't stop. I was addicted. The way addiction works, whether it's alcohol or heroin or food or sex, is that you latch onto a thing or a habit or a substance that gives you a reprieve from reality. But when more problems arise from the substance you're abusing, that substance then presents itself as the solution to the same problems it has caused. And round and round you go, not even recognizing the cycle you've created for yourself. It's only looking back now that I can see the pattern.

Addiction runs on shame, and my church taught me to be ashamed of sex. Shame tells you that you're bad by nature: In your sitting, resting mode, you're evil. Original sin—that's your default. You have to work and fight and pray and claw to be good, because being good is not your natural state. Anytime you do anything wrong, it's "Oh well, I guess this is who I really am." Then when you do something good, you say, "Okay, I went the extra mile. I want my cookie. I want my reward." And that reward is usually something bad. Which starts the cycle over again. You feel horrible about being bad, so you work hard to be good and then reward yourself by being bad until you feel so horrible you go out and do good. For some people it's alcohol. For others it's food. For me it was pornography. I'd go to the drugstore and buy the magazines, have them for a week or a month, throw them away in disgust, and then go buy more the minute I broke down again. After a while, I figured this was how my life was going to be and that it must be normal.

Because it was normal. Because everyone I knew, from my parents to my pastor, had a double life like me. I'd learned to play the game: Put the best foot forward. Paint the picture. Look righteous and decent and good. My outward appearances became more important than who I actually was. I became obsessed with achieving perfection in all areas of my life, to be so perfect that I could make up for the bad things I did in secret, or at least to make sure no one ever found out about them.

The thing about shame and addiction is that they will take you a long way. A double life works until it doesn't. The shame kicks you into a higher gear, and my shame absolutely did that for me. I was a super-high achiever, played every sport, voted Most Likely to Succeed, the whole thing. I'd get all these rewards and go, go, go, and then it would start to crumble and I'd completely fall apart and let myself go, all the while praying that no one would find out. It wasn't sustainable. It wasn't healthy. But I did get a lot done.

Overachieving looks good from the outside. People will always compliment you on it, and they'll never ask about whatever pathology is driving it. It wasn't enough to paint a picture that my teacher and classmates admired. I had to paint a picture that was flawless in every way. It wasn't enough to be good at sports. I had to be the best player of all time. It wasn't enough to behave in church. I had to be the best kid in the entire church. I started volunteering for everything. I volunteered for the solo in choir. I played the flute. I led the ceremony. If anyone needed anything, Terry Crews was ready, willing, and able. I wanted my image to be perfect because I wanted to make it to heaven. I wanted to get clean, but I would always find myself dirty again.

4

FOOL ME TWICE

When I was around eleven years old, right as I was coming of age and starting to hit puberty and dealing with this burgeoning addiction to porn, my mother called me into my bedroom, where she was sitting.

"Do you have hair down there yet?" she said.

"What?"

"Do you have hair down there?"

"Well, yeah, I guess?"

"Lemme see."

"Huh?"

"Pull your pants down. Lemme see."

"But, Trish . . ."

"Shut up. Do it."

So I did it. I pulled my pants down and stared out the window, trying not to meet her gaze. After what felt like forever she said, "Okay, fine. You can go play."

I pulled up my pants and ran outside and stayed outside all day, not wanting to come back in the house and saying to myself, "That didn't happen. That didn't happen. That didn't happen." Then I buried that memory as deep as I could, and it didn't resurface until I went into therapy thirty years later.

What she did that day was profoundly invasive and damaging. It was abusive in the sense of my feeling violated, and it was about control. It was about her reminding me, even as I was becoming a man, that I was still powerless because she was still the one in charge.

Religion made my mother cruel. When you live with so much guilt and shame all the time, you start to assume everyone around you is dirty and guilty, too. She was always suspicious of us, blaming us for things we didn't do. We were always guilty until proven innocent. Which is something that's true across all of America. Black men face horrible stereotypes at the hands of white people, but there's also a pervasive sentiment among some black women, from Oprah on down, that a lot of black men just ain't no good.

My mother's whole life had been derailed when some teenage boy got her pregnant. Now that she had two teenage boys of her own, forget it. She was sure we would get up to no good. Because of that, and because of church, we weren't allowed to date. I was not allowed to ask a girl to go anywhere, not to the movies or to the mall, nothing. Trish would always say, "God will give you the person you're supposed to get." And that was that. I would fight and argue with her about it all the time. "Why?" I'd say. "Why can't I go on a date?"

"Because you're stupid," she'd reply, "and you're going to get somebody pregnant. These girls are smarter than you."

She called me stupid a lot. That was her blanket answer for why I wasn't allowed to do anything. "Why can't I do it?" "Because you're stupid and you'll get in trouble." It was an insult that cut extra deep. Marcelle had struggled with real learning disabilities; he'd been held back a grade, and I'd seen the way people treated him because of it. To this day, if someone treats me like I'm less intelligent, or like I'm too dumb to follow what they're telling me, it makes me really, really angry. Because I hated it when my mother called me stupid.

She would still hit me, too. Even as I was bulking up in the gym and becoming a varsity football player, she'd smack me like I was still five years old. Usually I didn't let it get to me, but one time she whacked me, and before I could stop myself, I lifted my hand in the air, as a reflex. I was never going to hit her, and I was already lowering my hand when she snapped, "You raise your hand at me?" Big Terry happened to be walking into the room, and Trish turned to him with a wild look in her eye and said, "Terry, he was gonna hit me! He was gonna hit me!"

Big Terry started running after me and caught me at the stairs and tried to kick me. He missed and I looked back and he was howling in pain. He'd chipped a bone in his foot. Served him right. I left him on the stairs, went into my room, and shut the door. Staring out the window into the street, thinking about the wide world outside, all I could think was "I've got to get out of here. I've got to get out of this cult, and I've got to get out from under her."

Right before my high school graduation, there was an award ceremony for the departing seniors. I'd been voted Most Likely to Succeed, and I was being given the school's highest honor, the Spirit Award. My relationship with Big Terry and Trish had grown so acrimonious by that point that they didn't even come. I'd invited them, but they didn't show up. Maybe Trish wanted to teach me a lesson. Maybe Big Terry thought I'd gotten too full of myself. As I heard my name announced from the stage that night, I walked up to accept my plaque, and all I could think was "My parents aren't here to see this." I was so ready to go. I was fed up with my father's violence, fed up with my mother's hypocrisy. I got accepted to Western Michigan University, packed up my things, and moved down to Kalamazoo to go to college.

After a few months, I wound up joining another cult.

When I got to WMU, I was hopelessly naive. I was terrified of sex, terrified of being alone with a girl, terrified of alcohol. The first month of college, all the freshmen do is drink. They get that first taste of freedom and go crazy, which I thought I wanted, too. But I couldn't handle it. My suitemate had these keg parties. He'd put the keg in the bathroom and all these people would be in there getting wasted. The next morning, beer would be all over the floor, all sticky and nasty, and the smell reminded me of my father. I couldn't socialize with that crowd. And because I was a still a walk-on, I wasn't really part of the football team, either. I was all alone and needed a place to belong.

Even though I'd run screaming from my mother's cult, I was still the product of that cult. That dynamic felt comfortable to me. So when I was approached on campus by a representative of the Maranatha Christian ministry, I fell right back in to it. No cult presents itself to you as a cult. The people I met there were all warm and friendly, and it was a place to go instead of being alone on Friday night. Amid all this uncertainty and fear, it felt like home again. It's also true that I still had the mentality that "if you're a good person, you go to church." I truly thought faith was still the only thing that could make me do right and save me from the devil. So in the back of my mind, I was thinking, "I gotta keep my protection, just in case."

At first glance Maranatha seemed innocent enough, a campus spiritual group like any other, nothing involving a Charles Manson or a Jim Jones. Founded a few years earlier by a preacher named Bob Weiner and his wife, Rose, Maranatha was based in Gainesville,

Florida, and had branches on college campuses all over the country. I went to a couple of their services, and right away I was all in. Other than the familiarity of it, I got hooked because it appealed to my ego.

Maranatha's brilliance was in creating an aura of exclusivity. It actually called its members "God's Green Berets." Part of the recruiting process was giving you the names of all the successful people who'd come through Maranatha, and it was a real who's who of successful people from business and professional sports. The ministry wasn't a megachurch type of deal, either; every branch had only a few dozen members, and they recruited almost entirely from campus leader types and student athletes. The whole ethos was built around challenging you. "We want only quality people," they'd say. "This isn't for everyone. Giving yourself to Jesus isn't easy. Are you good enough to do what we're asking you to do? Are you ready to test yourself to see how far you can go? Are you the best of the best? Because Jesus wants only the best."

Which isn't actually true; it's pretty much the opposite of everything Jesus ever said about the last being first and the meek inheriting the earth. But it's an attractive concept for type A, goal-oriented people, which I was and still am. When I busted out of Flint, young and arrogant and telling myself I was destined for the NFL, Maranatha was right there waiting.

"Okay, Terry," they said. "You want to be the best?"

"Hell yeah, I want to be the best!"

"You think you have what it takes to be the best?"

"I *know* I got what it takes to be the best!"

"Okay. Here's what you have to do to be the best. Just follow all of these rules and do exactly what we say."

And they got me. Hook, line, and sinker. Unable and unwilling to confront my own weaknesses, I could see myself only as the dominant alpha male, and Maranatha used that to get me to make myself submit. It's a deviously brilliant technique, and it's something I'd see later in the culty, self-helpy, life-coachy movements that constantly pop up among the corporate CEO types of Hollywood and Silicon Valley and Wall Street.

The big saying at the core of Maranatha's teaching was "If Jesus is not Lord of all, then He's not Lord at all." Which is exactly the kind of simple sloganeering that cults use to get in your head. They get you to agree to one, broadly unobjectionable statement, and then use that as a Trojan horse to plant a bunch of bad ideas into your mind. Because what that slogan actually meant was that if you deny Jesus in any one part of your life, you're denying Jesus completely, which means you have to give Jesus (i.e., the cult) control over every aspect of your life. And slowly but surely, I did.

Being at college, I was all excited that I finally got to listen to secular music whenever I wanted. Then one night I was listening to the Beastie Boys in my dorm room, and one of the church members heard me.

"Hey, Terry," he said, leaning in my door. "What are you listening to?"

"This is the new Beastie Boys. It's really hot."

"Terry, you know you can't listen to that kind of stuff."

"What do you mean?'

"You love Jesus, right?"

"Yeah, of course."

"Well, you see Jesus has to be Lord of all or he's not Lord at all. And Jesus wouldn't listen to that music, so we can't listen to that music."

"Oh . . . oh, okay."

And I threw away my music, all my cassette tapes and my mixtapes of early hip-hop. Because I believed I had to make this commitment to God—and because I wasn't ready to be free. Freedom is scary if you don't know how to navigate it. I didn't know how to be autonomous and responsible for myself outside of this hyper-religious world of people telling me the rules I had to follow. So on the one hand I hated getting rid of my rap music, but on the other hand, getting rid of it felt like I was home again.

For the first year and a half of college, Maranatha became my whole world. I was so scared of all the drinking and partying that I didn't try to get to know anyone outside of the ministry. I didn't even make friends on the football team. It would have been bad enough if the only thing Maranatha had tried to control was my musical tastes and my choice of friends, but of course it didn't stop there. Every religion sets out to control your sex life, because if you control a person's sex life, you control that person entirely.

My pastor at Maranatha was a guy named Greg Dickow, who's now the pastor at the Life Changers megachurch outside of Chicago. He'd told me when I first joined that if I was thinking about dating a girl, I should talk to him first to make sure God wanted us to be together. That wasn't a problem for me, as I was so terrified of women that, up to that point, I had simply opted not to date at all.

Because my mom never allowed me to date, throughout high school the bad ideas I had about sex affected only one person: me. But now I was in college, living in a coed dorm. Temptation was right down the hall. Boys and girls were out sowing their wild oats. I now had to navigate the world of actual, three-dimensional women.

It went about as well as you might expect.

There's a reason that shame makes you cruel. It's because any slip, any sin, makes you feel terrible about yourself, so you go looking for someone else to blame for making you feel that pain. That was the reason for my mother's cruelty. With all her verbal and physical abuse, she was lashing out at whoever she felt led her away from God or into temptation. In her mind, that person was responsible for her pain. That person had revealed her weakness and was keeping her out of heaven. That cycle is bad enough for anyone in any context, but when it comes specifically to men and sex, when men are made to feel guilt and shame around sex, it makes them hate women, because they are the ones "tempting us" into sin. It's a story as old as Adam and Eve: she bids him to eat the apple, and the whole world falls from grace. *It's all her fault.*

Before I got to Western Michigan, I never would have thought of myself as a man who hated women. I was "the nice guy." Because I couldn't date in high school, I was also the safe guy, the sweet guy. My best friends were three white girls I ate lunch with every day. They were wonderful. But the women in the porn magazines, well, they weren't women. They weren't even people. They were objects.

The first time I came close to losing my virginity was a rainy day when a girl I knew came by my room. She was hanging around and flirting and giving me all kinds of signs, saying things like "Y'know, there are a lot of things you can do in the rain." Stuff like that. Believing I had to be righteous and keep myself clean, I resisted. I ignored her until she finally got the message and left. In my messed-up mind, I actually felt great about that. "You were good, Terry. You did good. You didn't let her ruin you."

Then, one night right before Christmas break, I was in my Zimmerman Hall dormitory room, feeling restless and low down, when I noticed a girl go into the room next door. I'd seen her around. We'd talk occasionally when we bumped into each other around the dorm. So I took a deep breath, put on a smile I didn't really feel, and walked over to her open doorway. "Hey, what's up?" I said.

"Hey, Terry," she said, smiling back at me.

"You busy?" I said.

She invited me in, and we both sat down on beanbags on the floor. Her roommate had already left for her winter break. We made small talk as usual, listened to Michael Jackson's "The Lady in My Life," and as time went on, it was clear that neither one of us wanted to go. The next thing I knew, we were kissing, and then we were both stretched out on the carpet. Even as it was happening, I felt like it was wrong, but I didn't stop. Finally, I was touching a real woman. This was my chance to see what sex was all about. So I did.

It was every bit as awkward and as terrible as you might imagine it would be, given how inexperienced I was. What was wild and strange and confusing about it was that I never climaxed. I couldn't get out of my own head, and I just went and went and went until I stopped because I didn't know what to do.

"What's wrong?" she said. "Did you finish?"

I didn't even know how to answer. I had to get out of there as soon as possible because of all the shame I felt being there. And because I felt that shame, I looked at her and I despised her, immediately. I wasn't a virgin anymore. She'd ruined me.

The minute it was over I wanted to leave. I'd gone against everything I'd been taught. I pulled on my clothes as quickly as I could, hardly looking at her as I ducked out of her room, thinking, *How did that happen? How did that happen? How did that happen?* For so long, I'd been waiting to have sex, and fantasizing about sex, and thinking about the kind of woman I wanted to marry and have sex with, and now it had finally happened, but it hadn't been at all like I'd wanted it to be. I was so disappointed, mostly in myself. I took a shower for what felt like an hour, trying to wash it all off.

In the weeks that followed, I fell into a spiral of self-righteousness, because I'd been taught that I was supposed to be better than people like her. I had myself up on a pedestal, and she'd knocked me off. The truly messed-up part was that now, because we'd slept together, even though I was consumed with feelings of hatred for her, I felt like I was supposed to date her. I needed to make it a relationship in order to retroactively make it right. We ended up seeing each other and sleeping together a few more times, and every time I felt horrible and I'd push her away again. It actually replaced my porn addiction for a while. I was using her the same way I used porn: go buy the magazines, act out, feel shame, throw the magazines away, and then go buy them again. Only now I was doing that to a person.

The situation was doubly toxic because she was not someone who was in a healthy place, either. She was dealing with some mental health and self-esteem issues of her own. The whole thing ended in a screaming fight in the hallway of the dorm. I was in the process of moving into another dorm anyway, and I used that as an excuse to walk away from the whole thing and pretend it had never happened.

Consumed by feelings of guilt, I went to Pastor Dickow for guidance. I wanted someone to pray with, to help me get back on the right path. When I spoke to him, I was so focused on being angry at myself that I didn't register the discomfiting ways he was pressing me for the intimate details of what had gone down. He was my pastor and he assured me I could speak to him in confidence, so I told him everything.

A few weeks later, right after New Year's, I joined Pastor Dickow and some of our other church members for a big conference of all the Maranatha campus ministries at the Omni hotel in Dallas, Texas. There were lots of events and speeches and convocations, and one of them was a speech that Rose Weiner, the "mother" of the church, was going to give to all the black members of the ministry. In terms of race, Maranatha was mixed. Mostly white, but it heavily recruited black kids, especially among student athletes. Rose Weiner, however, was *very* white, and when she took to the podium to give her speech to all the black students, she said, "We have to be grateful for the love of God, and for Christianity, and for all of you being saved, because if it weren't for Christianity, all of you would be worshipping idols in the jungle."

You could almost hear a collective snap as every head in the room whipped around simultaneously to stare at her. The same expression was on every face, too: "Oh, she did *not* just say that."

I couldn't believe it. I sat there, trying so hard to process what she'd said that I couldn't pay attention to another word she spoke. Once she was done, Brett Fuller, one of Maranatha's few black ministers, took over the stage. Brett is currently the senior pastor of Grace Covenant Church in Virginia along with being the chaplain for the NFL's Washington, DC, team.

"Now," he said, "you all know we needed to hear that."

"Nope," I thought. "I did not need to hear that at all. The Kool-Aid may have gotten to you, brother. But not to me."

I went back to the hotel where we were all staying, and someone from our ministry told me that Pastor Dickow wanted to talk to me down in one of the conference rooms. I walked into the room, but instead of Pastor Dickow waiting for me alone, he was there with ten other Maranatha preachers. They were sitting in a semicircle, with one single chair in the middle, as if it were some kind of tribunal. One of the pastors gave me a hard look.

"We heard about your infidelity," he said.

"I told them about what you did," Pastor Dickow said. "And now we're going to get over this together. These men are going to help you to overcome your demons."

Incredulous, I looked at Pastor Dickow. I sat down slowly, feeling as naked as the day my mother made me expose myself to her. I already felt horrible about what I'd done, and this only made it worse because now I'd been betrayed. I'd trusted my pastor to keep my secrets in confidence, and here he'd told everyone and dragged me into a public shaming. One at a time, they all lit into me, telling me I'd done wrong

"Terry, you know this was wrong, right?" one said. "Sexual sin is something that will take you out for the rest of your life."

"You were representing this church," another said. "You are one of our leaders, and you cannot behave in this way."

When it was over, Dickow looked at me with a smug expression and said, "You needed that."

After what the church "mother" had said, and now this, I knew what I needed was to get the hell away from these people. We drove back to Kalamazoo, and I didn't say a word the whole trip. I didn't show up for the next meeting or the one after that or the one after that. I started getting phone calls from different members of our church, telling me all of the scary stuff that was going to happen to me if I left. But I didn't care. The scales had fallen from my eyes. I'd seen enough to know that Maranatha, despite its trappings, was no different from the cult my mother had raised me in. I was out. But instead of feeling elated that I'd stood up for myself, I was devastated. Because I was alone again.

The people I thought were my friends excommunicated me. They decided, "He won't be a part of our church, so we won't talk to him." And because I'd joined a church group that looked down on our classmates as sinners, I'd never made any other friends; I'd allowed the church to isolate me on campus the same way my mother had isolated us from our family back in Flint. For the next few weeks, I was like a zombie. I was the loneliest I've ever been. I was almost tempted to go back to Maranatha, just to be around people. It was harder to be alone than it was to be with people I knew were exploiting me. But I knew I couldn't. After being at school and on the football team for nearly two years, I found myself starting over, because I'd been there but I hadn't been there. I had to walk up to my teammates in the locker room and my neighbors in the dorm and say, "Hey, I'm Terry."

About a month or so after leaving Maranatha, I found one guy from my dorm to hang out with. His name was Joseph Applewhite. He was at Western Michigan on a track scholarship for the long jump; this brother could leap and fly like a gazelle. He'd been to a Maranatha meeting and decided it wasn't for him, so he understood what I'd been through. He was the only person I could talk to about what had happened. He had a girlfriend, April, and they were good people, a lifeline for me. They took me on as their little project and would always include me in whatever they were doing. At times I felt like a third wheel, but I was so lonely I didn't care.

Then one day Joe and April invited me to go with them to their own church, Christian Life Center, for their Wednesday night service. Nervous about dipping my toe back into those waters, I decided to go anyway. The church itself was a small, traditional-looking white chapel on Kalamazoo's north side. We walked in, and that familiar church smell of Pine-Sol hit me, bringing back all sorts of memories. But what really struck me was the music. It wasn't churchy at all. It had a nice groove that made me bop my head.

Then I saw the pianist. She was bowed over the keys of a late-model synthesizer like Schroeder from *Peanuts*, only she was beautiful. She had short, curly, sandy-brown hair with scattered blond highlights. Skinny, too, with olive skin and an exotic look about her. Whatever her ethnicity was, I couldn't guess it from across the room, and I was curious about how she fit in with the mostly black congregation. As the service began, she got up from the keyboard and sat a few rows ahead of me.

It felt good to be there, away from the dormitory and its raucous, juvenile behavior, in a place that felt clean, like everyone in the room was trying to be a better person. The sermon was okay, but I don't remember much of it because I spent most of the time stealing glances over at the piano player.

When I went to leave at the evening's end, Joe held me back. "There's someone I want you to meet," he said. Then he reached up his arm and waved over the piano player. Right as she started walking in our direction, someone handed her a blond baby. "Oh," I thought. "She's a mother. Maybe she's the pastor's wife. So much for that." But then she kept walking over with a small baby planted firmly on her hip, and Joe said, "Rebecca, this is my friend, Terry. Terry, this is Rebecca."

She smiled and extended her free hand to me. I shook it and did my best to make small talk as my mind raced to try to figure out what her story was. Her story was that she was an unmarried single mother, living on her own. She worked in a hair salon and played piano on the side and, despite my initial confusion about her appearance, she was black.

Over the next few weeks, Joe and April kept bringing me along on different outings, and Rebecca was usually there; the whole Wednesday night church invitation had been a ruse to set the two of us up. Given who I was and where I was in my life at the time, it never should have worked out. I was still walking the tightrope of guilt and shame around sex. My porn addiction and my double life were as crippling and debilitating as ever. I was in no way mature enough to fully understand and appreciate her. If Rebecca had been a fully formed, all-together person, she would have taken one look at me and realized, "There's no way I can be with this clown." But she and I were both broken in our own ways. It turned out that we needed each other, not just as man and wife, but as people—two human beings, two souls lost in the universe who happened to stumble upon one another.

As I got to know Rebecca better, and learned more about her situation, both my sympathy and admiration for her increased. She was definitely more mature than I was, but she was going through a lot.

Growing up in Gary, Indiana, her father had died when she was six, and she'd had a nervous breakdown in high school. She still went on to win the Miss Gary pageant in 1984 and become a musical theater major with a 4.0 grade point average. But that's when she got pregnant. She hadn't been dating the baby's father, and she'd considered giving her baby up for adoption but couldn't do it. When it became clear the father was incapable of helping to raise the child, Rebecca dropped out of college and went on food stamps and subsidized housing while she completed beauty school. She was in a very vulnerable position.

In our mutual brokenness, we fell almost right away into a kind of interdependence. Neither of us had any money, but she had a subsidized apartment we could share, and I had a car she could use to get to work. If we pooled our resources, we could almost make a complete life together. That kind of symbolized where we both were emotionally as well: I'm incomplete and you're incomplete, but maybe together we make a whole. And despite my staggering immaturity, there was voice inside of me wise enough to understand that this woman was the person I needed to be with. I had a feeling and sense that we were connected. There was something that we were supposed to do together. I didn't even know what it was.

The fact that she had a baby was a huge obstacle for to me; I was in no way ready for a family. But on one of our first big dates, I looked at her and said, "Y'know, I don't know where this is going to go, but I want you to know that I'm willing." I hadn't even planned on saying it; it just came out. We tied the knot one year later. It would take another twenty years for us both to reckon with our brokenness and find our way to a truly healthy marriage, but in the moment, all we knew for sure was that we loved each other and we needed each other, and we had to hope that that would be enough.

5

ROCK BOTTOM

After Maranatha, I decided I would never again give myself over to any religious organization. To this day I have an allergic reaction to it. It's visceral. Anytime I hear gospel music, I can feel myself getting angry as the dark memories come flooding back. I hate any kind of choir music; when gospel singers come on *America's Got Talent*, I literally have to stop and remind myself to evaluate them on their merits and not let my own bad experiences get in the way.

Unfortunately, right after I made my vow never to set foot in a church again, I met my future wife . . . at church. Rebecca was religious. It was especially important to her to raise her kids in the church, and if her church had been anything like the Holy Roller nonsense I grew up with, I couldn't have done it. I would have turned around and walked out, and we never would have gotten married. Fortunately, she had grown up Methodist, where the services were very staid and calm. Nobody dancing or running up and down the aisles. The Christian Life Church she attended with Joe and April was nondenominational, but it was in that vein as well. It was sober, reasonable people coming together for the positive things religion ought to bring, like moral instruction and community. That I could handle, so I set my issues aside and went back.

After we got married, I began my wandering years in the NFL, moving from LA to San Diego to DC. In every city, Rebecca would find a church she wanted the family to attend, and I would go, too. For her and for the kids. Never for myself. I'd put on my suit and go to the services and the picnics and the fundraisers and smile and be friendly. It was a nice way to meet new people in a strange town and give the kids some Sunday school lessons in right and wrong. But that was it. Inside, I always kept the whole thing at arm's length.

Still, at the same time, I always kept the door open. I never became full-on atheist, or even an agnostic. I still see the world in a very spiritual, emotional way. Even as a kid, and nothing to do with my mom's church, I had always viewed myself as a soul within a body. I've always felt that I didn't create myself, that there is more to our existence than what we can see and touch, that there is a purpose to our lives beyond mere survival. I look at the world and I'm full of questions. I'm always trying to connect my own dots with all the crazy stuff I've seen. I loved taking physics in college, because physics is the science of trying to imagine what's not there. Honestly, I think religion stifled that in me to a large degree. Religion—at least the religion I was exposed to—only tells you "this is how it is." The further I got away from that, the better I felt. By the time we settled in LA, with Maranatha in my rearview and my church attendance largely reduced to a social obligation, I felt like my spiritual life was vastly improved, because I wasn't being spoon-fed the answers. I had to search for them myself. So I thought I was good. I wasn't.

Old habits die hard. Which we now know isn't simply a matter of willpower. Unhealthy behaviors literally get wired into the physical neural pathways in our brain, like deeply grooved, well-worn paths we can't get out of. That's how it was for my mother. She finally saw the light enough to leave Elder Jones and Greater Holy Temple Church of God in Christ, but she was so accustomed to this pattern of being told what to do that she always ended up back in the clutches of some strange new outfit, like I had with Maranatha. The one she finally ended up with was a thing called Faith Tech. It was a small group of mostly women who met in a community center where they would sit and read the Bible and other spiritual works. Their whole thing was "We're going to come up with our own revelations from Jesus!" I heard that and was like, "Uh-oh." I didn't even want to know what kind of Kool-Aid drinking was going on there. It was like a cross between a cult and a book club. It was very Oprah. They all loved Oprah.

Unfortunately, I hadn't left that world behind as much as I liked to think I had. I'd rejected the institutions of it, but those institutions had shaped who I was. They had made me into a person driven to succeed at all costs and live behind a veneer of overachieving perfection, a person whose every action was governed by fear and shame and guilt, particularly with regard to sex. I had no internal moral compass of my own. The only reason I knew to do right was to earn some kind of reward. The only reason I knew not to do wrong was to avoid getting caught. So underneath this self-righteous facade of acting as if I were better than everyone else, all my bad habits and my addictive, self-destructive behaviors continued.

Unsurprisingly, my addiction to pornography waxed and waned depending on how the rest of my life was going at the time. All through my NFL years, if I was killing it on the field and feeling successful, I could go weeks or even months without using it. But the moment my stress levels spiked, from the fear of getting cut from a team or the anxiety of not knowing if I'd get re-signed, I would reach for it again. I would go and get magazines from liquor stores and then throw them away. If I was on the road, I'd order pay-per-view movies in my hotel room.

The arrival of the internet made everything worse. The first iMacs came out right around the time I left the NFL and we had moved to LA so I could try to break into the entertainment business. Once we brought a computer into the house, it was the same as when I'd made the leap from magazines to late-night cable. Everything escalated. These were the days of dial-up, so it took half an hour to load an image, but now there was no more sneaking out to video stores to get a fix. It was all right there at the touch of a button. It also became easier not to leave a trail of evidence. Just delete the images and the search history and no one would be the wiser.

Then, in 1999, my addiction made its most dangerous leap yet. Having gone from the page to the television to the computer, it crossed over into the real world. After appearing on TV in the reality gladiator show *Battle Dome*, I'd landed my first serious acting job in the Arnold Schwarzenegger movie *The 6th Day*, which was shooting in Vancouver over the course of five months. That movie was the door opening to my dream of working in movies. It was also the first good money I'd made since professional football: $75,000 for five months of work, plus $600 a week in per diem. With the exchange rate from the US to Canada being what it was, it was like Monopoly money. There was no way I wasn't doing this job, but I was miserable. I was completely overwhelmed. After one season on a reality show, I was playing one of the henchmen in an $80 million Schwarzenegger tentpole action movie. I didn't need to stay in Vancouver the whole five months, but I was scared to leave, thinking if I wasn't around and available, they might decide they didn't need me as much. Or they might even realize I was no good and fire me. Being on that set gave me the worst anxiety I've ever experienced. I felt like this was my one shot. I couldn't afford to blow it. I'd been cut so many times in the NFL, I was always afraid of it happening again.

Because I didn't know my castmates that well, and I was around them only when we filmed, I was always alone. I didn't know what I was doing, and I was constantly racked with self-doubt. My refuge from the anxiety and doubt, as always, was porn. Being at home had always put guardrails on my addiction. I didn't want Rebecca to find it in the house, didn't want to run into anybody I knew at the video store or a seedy movie theater. But my hotel had a full supply of pornographic movies I could order right in my room. I watched all of them. Some of them twice. There were times when I wasn't needed on set for weeks. I would work out in the morning and be alone in my room for the rest of the day. It was the worst-case scenario for someone like me.

One Friday night I was looking through Vancouver's alt-weekly newspaper for a movie to go see, and in the back were all these ads for massage parlors. They had pictures of scantily clad women on them, the suggestion being that this place offered much more than a massage. I'd been in Vancouver for a couple of months by that point and, having run out of porn to watch on the hotel TV, I told myself I needed a massage from all the working out I'd been doing. I got in my rental car to go and "take a look."

I went to the address that was in one of the ads. It was not on the nice side of town. Vancouver had a huge drug problem for a long time, and the addicts were out in force. I drove up and parked, walked back and forth past the entrance several times, but then finally went in. There were women seated and lined up against the wall in lingerie-style clothing. I want to say there were about ten of them, all different races and ethnicities. I told the female receptionist I was there for a massage, and she told me to pick one of the ladies. I know for a fact I picked the one who made eye contact with me, because the rest of them mostly sat there in a lifeless daze.

The receptionist brought me back to a room and told me to put on a robe and wait. I was so nervous. I knew I had no business being there. Everything inside me was screaming "GET OUT!" but I kept moving through it, telling myself, lying to myself, that it would just be a massage.

The woman came in and asked me what I wanted. I told her I wanted a massage. Did I want the regular, the deluxe, or "the special"? I shrugged because I couldn't bring myself to say it. She told me the prices for each and I gave her cash for the most expensive one. She took the money and nodded like, "Let's get this over with." After a few minutes of going through the motions with the "therapeutic massage," she turned me over and gave me a hand job. Then she asked when I would come back, gave me a card with a number on it, and told me to ask for her. I took it, got dressed, and left as fast as I could. I never went back.

When I got to my room, the full weight of what I'd done began to sink in. I had done the unthinkable: I'd cheated on my wife. Rebecca was at home excited that I was in another country doing a job people dream about, finally seeing the results of all our sacrifice, but instead I was here watching porn and cheating on her with a stranger. The world seemed to close in on me, and everything was super dark. The shame rushed in all at once, and there was no escape. For the first time in my life, I had intense suicidal thoughts. I put my head in my hands and cried all night.

On Sunday I drove to a church way out in the suburbs, and after the service, I went up to the altar, got on my knees, and cried in front of this strange congregation. I'm sure they were wondering what my story was, but I damn sure wasn't about to tell it. I went back to my room from that service and vowed that no one would ever know what happened at that massage parlor. I would take this secret to my grave, no matter what.

The rest of that shoot was a dark time, and it only got darker. Although acting out had alleviated my stress in the moment, it had done nothing to help me with my guilt and shame in the long term. I was still lonely, homesick, and worried I might get fired at any moment. Only now it was worse because I was afraid to go home and face my wife.

I made it to the end of the shoot and flew back to LA, and for a long time this secret ate away at my conscience. But Rebecca never found out. The Rapture didn't come down and rain God's judgment upon me, and because there hadn't been any punishment, I was able to tell myself it hadn't been that bad. I put it out of my mind and blocked it out so completely that I didn't think about it at all. I never cheated on Rebecca again, but I didn't break out of my addiction to pornography, either. Having endured the shame of going further than porn, I was able to convince myself that the porn habit was actually not that bad. I was staying faithful. I was doing the right thing. Plus, everyone else watched porn, too. Everyone else had a double life, too. I was just doing what everyone else was doing. I was one of the good guys, right?

6

D-DAY

On February 6, 2010, my marriage and my life finally came crashing down around me. I was on location in New York City, holed up in my hotel room as a huge snowstorm battered the windows outside. Rebecca and I were arguing on the phone, which we'd been doing a lot lately. After the forty-year high-wire act of holding myself together, I was finally coming apart. Inside, I was a mess, less a person and more a collection of barely controlled compulsions and habits: a simmering cauldron of rage born of the powerlessness I felt in the face of just about everything. I was a liar, an addict, a dirty, shameful sinner.

Outwardly, I was compensating for all of that with my pathological need for control. I was trying to control things I had no business trying to control, like my wife and children, and things I couldn't control even if I'd wanted to, like the course of my career in Hollywood. I was driven not merely by a desire to have the perfect life, but by an obsessive need to show the whole world how perfect it was. So much so that I'd talked my wife and kids into joining me for *The Family Crews*, a reality show on BET. For months, cameras had been following us around and documenting how wonderful our life was, when it was anything but.

Meanwhile, the anxiety of holding everything together was fraying my last nerve. I was walking around short tempered, agitated. I had no idea what was actually wrong with me. I had everything I'd ever worked for—the beautiful wife, the successful career, the nice house, the fancy car—and I wasn't happy at all. And for the life of me I couldn't understand why.

Rebecca knew something was wrong. For months she'd been saying, "Terry, what's going on? There's something you're not telling me." As she said it again that night on the phone in my hotel room, I thought to myself, "Terry, this is your chance. She knows. If you tell her now, you'll probably lose her. But if you don't tell her now, you'll definitely lose her, because she'll know that you're lying. Either way, at least this is a chance for you to actually get clean."

So I came clean. The massage parlor in Vancouver, the years of pornography addiction—I told her everything. She broke down crying. I felt like I'd shot her in the chest. We sat there on the phone, and she cried and cried. "You've been lying to me for ten years?" she said. "And you put me on television, knowing that you did this? How *could* you?"

She told me not to come home, that I needed to find another place to live, and I understood. In that moment, I thought I'd lost it all. My fancy hotel room felt like a prison cell. I sat there in the dark, the winter storm howling outside, with no idea what to do with myself. I needed help. I needed guidance. More than anything I needed someone to talk to. So I picked up the phone and did something a younger version of me never would have considered.

I called my pastor.

Rebecca and I had tried a few different churches after settling in Los Angeles. Anything that carried a whiff of Church of God in Christ back in Flint, I couldn't handle at all. If I heard any preacher get up and start with all that hootin' and hollerin', I'd immediately be like, "I'm out!" Ultimately, we ended up at a place called Faith Community in West Covina. It was a megachurch in terms of its size, for sure. Maybe seven or eight thousand people. But it didn't have the cultish feel that so many megachurches do. They did a lot of good for the community, Fourth of July picnics and barbecues for the homeless. It was all volunteer, and I never felt any pressure. At the cultish churches, you miss a Sunday or two and then you show up and people are like, "Where were you last week?" Forget that. At Faith Community it was nothing but smiles and "Hey, good to see you!" You showed up when you wanted to show up, and when you didn't show up, nobody was on you about it. That's all I wanted.

The pastor was a guy named Jim Reeve, and he and I had a good relationship. He didn't have an ounce of Elder Jones in him. He was a Southern California white guy, very feel good-y, very nondenominational, not judgmental at all. He didn't use religion to condemn or coerce anyone. He never had any problems with any of the R-rated work I was doing in the movies, either. He even came to a couple of my premieres.

Still, as much as I liked the pastor and the people and the charity work we did there, I was still of the mind that church was something I did only for my wife and kids. If it wasn't for them, I wouldn't even bother. But when I found myself in my darkest moment, I didn't know who else to call. I *had* no one else to call. Nobody in my life knew about all the darkness I was carrying inside me. I'd kept it all buttoned up behind this perfectionist facade, and I was too ashamed to tell anyone the truth. But I knew I could tell Pastor Reeve. I called him from New York, and I told him everything.

"What do I do?" I said. "I'm going to lose her."

"At the very least," he said, "stick to your normal routine. If your plan was to work out tomorrow morning, go work out tomorrow morning. Don't wallow in this. Keep moving forward so you don't disintegrate."

Then he gave me the advice that changed my life. "Terry," he said. "I cannot promise you that you're going to get your wife back or your family back. They may be gone forever, and that's her choice to make. But what you need to understand is that, whether she comes back or not, you need to get better for you."

"What do you mean?" I said.

"I mean that you don't need to just get better so that she'll come back to you. You need to get better for you."

His point was that virtuous behavior is not a means to an end, but an end itself. That was a watershed moment for me. My whole life, I'd had no internal moral compass of my own, no sense of doing right for its own sake. A true and benevolent religion, as opposed to a cult, might have given that to me. But the Church of God in Christ hadn't. My only sense of morality was based on a system of punishment and reward. You did good in life to avoid punishment and receive rewards, but you were never good for the sake of being good.

I recently came across a quote that sums up everything about my childhood experience with religion. It's a saying that goes "By gifts we make slaves, and by whips we make dogs." That's how the Church of God in Christ operated. With one hand it gave us gifts, like salvation and the only social connections and earthly pleasures we were allowed to have. With the other hand it whipped us and beat us with fear and guilt and, above all, shame.

All I knew how to do in life was to beg for the gifts and avoid the whip. I never learned how to be a good person simply for the fact that living a virtuous life is simply the better, healthier way to live. I ran screaming from my mother's cult and from Maranatha, thinking I'd left it all behind, thinking I was *better* than all those people who still went every Sunday and lived their lives as hostages to that stuff. But I was still a hostage myself. I'd never actually been deprogrammed from what the cult had taught me. I'd learned it so well that not only did I live my life that way, I treated my loved ones that way, too. I used gifts to control them. I would buy my kids the toys they wanted, or a car on their sixteenth birthday, and then I'd use that as leverage to lay down all my expectations of how I wanted them to behave. When that didn't work, I'd pull out the whip: my temper. It was rule by an iron fist. My way or the highway. I still ask my older daughters for their forgiveness to this day. We've got a lot of healing left to do, and that's all because of me. Luckily, with my younger kids and especially with my son, I've learned to set the gifts and the whips aside and parent with empathy and understanding instead, because I know now that's how I wish someone had treated me.

The nine-year-old me who stumbled across that trunk of dirty magazines in my uncle John's basement had nothing to be ashamed of. I was a normal kid with normal sexual curiosity. I was also an abused and traumatized kid looking for a release and an escape from the pain of the world I grew up in. I didn't need to be shamed for that. I didn't need to be whipped for that. I needed my parents to stop the cycle of abuse in our home. I needed a family therapist to lead me to a healthier understanding of sex and the compulsions I was experiencing, to arrest the cycle of addiction before it began. I didn't get that, not until I was a fully grown, forty-two-year-old man who was so damaged I'd been hurting the people who loved me for years.

Slowly, Rebecca and I began talking again. She opened the door for forgiveness and reconciliation, with the nonnegotiable stipulation that I get professional help. The next month, I entered a one-week program for sex addiction at a place called Psychological Counseling Services in Arizona. I was willing to do whatever it took to save my marriage, but even as I was checking into the facility, I was still telling myself, "This is crazy. I'm not like these people. Maybe I went too far with the massage parlor, and it got me here, but that's it. I mean, come on. What man doesn't look at pornography?"

It was only after I began talking to my counselors and attending group sessions that I began to understand that most men didn't have the same problems and compulsions that I did. I wasn't "watching" it. I was addicted to it. I started to see the patterns, how I always resorted to porn whenever I was nervous, stressed, or angry. The counselors actually had an acronym for it: HALT (hungry, angry, lonely, tired). If an addict is feeling any of these emotions, those are the times when he's most likely to slip. So I learned to examine my feelings and create new triggers for healthier behaviors.

For the rest of the week, it was one epiphany after another, and that week was the catalyst that blew open the doors to my examining and changing every aspect of my life.

Letting go of my shame-based morality and being led by my own internal moral compass changed the way I looked at everything and everyone. I understand the ways in which living with shame fueled my rage and my temper. I used to fly off the handle at people for the slightest lapse or imperfection, and it was because I was always mad at myself for the slightest lapse or imperfection. Living with shame made me cruel the same way it made my mother cruel. Like Trish, I was so self-righteous, judging people by the same impossible standard I was using to judge myself. Every time I broke down and used pornography, it meant I was weak and pathetic and worthless. I thought my failings were purely a matter of willpower, so every time I failed, I hated myself for failing. Which is why I used to look at alcoholics and say they were weak. I used to look at fat people and say they were lazy. I was that guy, and everybody hates that guy.

Now that I understand that that's not true for me, I know that it's not true for anyone. Learning to live without shame gave me genuine empathy for the first time. I look at every person in the world, and I understand that we've all got issues and we're all in the process of *becoming*. If someone hasn't vanquished their demons, or doesn't know how to vanquish their demons, or isn't even aware that they have demons to vanquish—I get it, because I lived that way for the first forty-two years of my life, and I've been unlearning it every day for the last ten.

In 2021, pornography is more ubiquitous than at any other time in human history. You don't have to go through four years of flute lessons to get it anymore. It's right there at the click of a button, twenty-four hours a day. And I've never been better. It plays no part in my life anymore, because I've escaped the shame-fueled cycle that had me addicted to it. I learned to live without shame. I don't hide my failings anymore. I operate in a lane of full disclosure.

Once I came clean and told Rebecca and my pastor and my therapist, I *felt* clean. Telling people, letting it all out there, felt so good. And what felt even better was telling the world. A few years later, Facebook Live was rolled out as a service on the platform. I was in my car testing it out, and as I was talking, I said, "Screw it," and I put it all out there. I talked about my addiction to pornography to all of Facebook. I made a statement that was raw and from the heart and wasn't practiced at all. "For years, years, years, my dirty little secret was that I was addicted to pornography," I said, "and it really, really messed up my life in a lot of ways. I didn't tell anybody. I didn't tell my wife. And the thing that I found is that by not telling people, it became more powerful. But when you tell everyone, when you put it out to the world like I'm doing right now, it loses its power." I laid out the history of what Rebecca and I had been through, and then I concluded by saying, "It's never enough to ask forgiveness. You also have to make amends. You have to do whatever you can to help. So if you're going through some things like this, share with me. Come with me. I want to help people. It's my mission. It's my life. It's what I do."

It went viral, instantly, and the next day, all the news shows wanted me on. *Good Morning America* was offering to fly me to New York. I told them, "Go watch the Facebook Live. It's all on there."

My publicist was flipping out. My agents were flipping out. It looked for a moment like the disclosure might cost me my sponsorship with Old Spice. For a day or two, people at the company were saying, "We gotta let him go." But then they didn't. Because they understood that I hadn't done anything wrong. I'd just been honest about my failings as a person—because I didn't have anything to be ashamed of. I still don't. My life is an open book.

In fact, you're reading it right now.

III

VALUE

1

FOR LOVE OR MONEY

Our house in Flint Park had rats. Lots and lots of rats. There were holes along the baseboards, too. So we had a ritual. My mother loved to watch *The Twilight Zone*, and every Friday night before *The Twilight Zone* came on, she'd set out traps with a piece of Kraft singles on them. Then we'd go watch our Friday night shows and, while we watched, one by one, the traps would go off.

Whap!

"Yeah! We got one!"

Whap! Whap!

"Oh! That's two more!"

We treated it like a game. Then, after the shows, my brother and I would have to clean the traps, which was not like a game at all. My mother would give us each a pair of our father's church socks, and we would put them on our hands and go and pull the dead rats out of the traps and throw them away. We'd do that until it was time to go to bed. It was wild.

When you're a kid, your reality is your reality. Whatever that is, it's normal to you. You don't know that, if you had more money, you wouldn't have rats in the first place. You don't know that you're poor. For me, wearing pants and shirts that were too small months after I'd outgrown them, that was normal. Eating all the groceries a day or two after going to the store and then having to wait for next Friday's paycheck to get more, that was normal.

Normal was my father trying to fix a broken heating pipe in my bedroom and watching millions of termites come pouring out of the wall like water from a faucet. That one was crazy. My dad panicked and made us run and put on our church shoes, the ones with the hard heels, and stomp them in the carpet. We kept stomping them and stomping them while he went to the store and got bug spray—the toxic kind, which was the only kind you could get back in the day. Then he came home and sprayed it all over our bedroom, and we had to sleep in there for days after. It was only when I got older and started going over to the houses of my friends and saw their nice furniture and their rat-free baseboards that I understood: "Oh, we don't have any money."

On top of my father's violent alcoholism and my mother's abusive personality, poverty was yet another reason why I had to put Flint in my rearview. It was also the reason I didn't follow my dream on the way out. Football was not my dream. What I loved was art. Visual art. Painting, sketching, sculpting. I'd started drawing when Marcelle went off to kindergarten, leaving me home alone with Trish all day. To keep me busy, she'd set out crayons and pencils on our brown wooden coffee table. I'd grab a pencil and kneel over the paper and let my imagination take over. Drawing was cathartic. I could visualize a different kind of world and escape to it. I could control what happened on the page or the canvas the way I couldn't control anything in life. I had the talent and the aptitude for it, too. Starting in elemen-

tary school, all of my teachers had nurtured that talent. My high
school art teacher, Mr. Eichelberg, used to tell me I was the best student he'd ever had. Even my father—a man who rarely took notice of
anything his children were doing—used to look at my drawings and
paintings and say, "Boy, you're like a Michelangelo right there!"

That was my dream, to be an artist. I loved movies and pop culture as much as fine art and dreamed of becoming an animator or a
set designer on films. I was talented enough to follow that path if I
wanted to, but by senior year, my parents had already told me, "You
ain't got no money for college. We're tryin' to put it together, but
don't go gettin' your hopes up."

The place I wanted to go to college was the Center for Creative
Studies in Detroit, but there was no way they were going to give me
a full ride. They didn't have a football team, so that meant no football scholarship, either. If I went there, I would need to pay my own
tuition, and that wasn't going to happen.

Even if I did get through college somehow, the idea of making a
living as an artist felt like a million-to-one shot. When I looked at
the world of art, even at the more practical professions like advertis-
ing and graphic design, I saw no one who looked like I did, no one
who came from where I came from. The only black man I'd ever even
heard of who was an artist was J. J. from *Good Times*, and he was a
fictional character—and as talented as J. J. was, the dude was still
stuck in the projects.

As crazy as it sounds, becoming a professional football player felt
like the more "practical" option. So I gave up on my dreams and followed the money. I gave up on the Center for Creative Studies and
walked on at Western Michigan to fight for my big ticket to the NFL.

But here's the thing: It never had to be that way. Because we
weren't actually poor.

2

GUESS WHERE
THE MONEY IS?

All my memories of childhood involve us having no money. My mother bouncing checks and juggling Peter to pay Paul, and always with the constant refrain of "We don't have it. We don't have it. We don't have it." But we did have it. We just didn't keep it. My father had a job, a good job. He was a foreman, a management-level position with General Motors, one of the largest and richest corporations in the world. For a black man in the 1970s who'd grown up with nothing in Jim Crow Georgia, my father had done well for himself. But he drank, and he gambled. And that's where the money went.

My dad always played the numbers. He played the legal one, the state lotto, and the illegal one, too. (The illegal lotto was a guy who took side bets on the state lotto. He was always coming around the barbershop with his little notebook, taking everyone's wagers.) My dad was in so deep it was never just a fun game for him. He had all these "strategies" that were going to help him win, as if it weren't all a scam to begin with. My dad even had a book that told you what numbers you should pick based on what dreams you had. He never asked about what my interests were or what I'd done at school that day, but he was always asking me, "What did you dream about last night?" If I told him "I saw a pig and it was flying," he'd look up "pig" and the book would say it meant you should pick thirty-nine. So he'd write that down and run off to give it to the numbers guy. I used to get so bored with it I'd make stuff up to bullshit him. "I dreamt I was on a cloud," I'd say, "and I reached down and threw a lightning bolt!" His eyes would widen, and he'd go, "Whoa! Lightning?!" Then he'd go to his little book and look up "lightning."

On the rare occasions he won, he'd put on a big celebration. He'd go out and get pizza, and then, on his way home, he'd take the money and hide it in different parts of his coats and his pants. Whenever I smelled pizza coming in the front door, I knew he'd won the numbers. He would come in shouting "I won! I won!" and then invite my mom and me and my brother and sister to play a game. "Guess where the money is! Guess where the money is!" We'd go into his shirt pocket or his coat pockets and pull out all the money. Whatever we didn't find, he'd take it out and throw it in the air, going, "I won! I won! Yeah!"

It didn't take me long to realize that even if you won a couple of times a year, if you were betting twenty or thirty dollars a day, you were never going to come out ahead. I even tried to tell him that. "Big Terry," I said, "this doesn't add up." But he wouldn't hear any of it.

My mother was as bad with money as he was, only she would do sweepstakes and contests. She entered all of them. She was always clipping those forms out of magazines and newspapers, licking stamps to mail them in. "This is how God's going to bless us," she'd say.

The upside of the sweepstakes and the contests was that, unlike playing the numbers, at least they didn't cost anything to enter. It wasn't money out of our pocket. Trish hated my dad's gambling because it was basically like setting money on fire. Not to mention the fact that we were told time and again at church that gambling was a sin. It was the devil getting in your money.

My mom was always on Big Terry about the gambling, but at the same time she would say stuff like, "Terry, I hope you get rich and get me out of here and buy me a house and we never have to come back here again." Whenever he won, she would play the money game right along with him. She'd dance and pull the money out and say, "Oh, God blessed us tonight!" So apparently it's the devil when you lose, but it's God when you win.

Eventually, my mom's sweepstakes mentality governed her entire approach to life. We weren't going to get out of poverty through hard work and responsibility. That was never a talk that we had. Instead, there was going to be some big lucky windfall that was going to come along and be our salvation. She even treated her kids like we were another sweepstakes. "One of y'all is gonna hit it big," she'd say. Every Sunday in the spring and summer we used to do the parade of homes after church. We'd go over to the nice side of town for the open houses of all the nice big homes for sale. We'd walk through, and she'd be like, "Ohhhh, these people got everything. This is what I want. I can't wait for you to grow up and get rich and get me one of these." So that became the expectation on all of us. Once I started getting noticed for playing ball, it was mostly on me.

It wasn't only my mom and dad who were terrible about money. It was the whole town of Flint. General Motors was, for a long time, a good company to work for. Too good, in some respects. Of course we should expect a company to pay its employees well and provide good benefits. But if you worked at the shop, as it was called, GM took care of *everything*. They gave you a car, financed your mortgage. It was damn near cradle to grave. So much so that even someone who drank and gambled as much as my father could still keep a roof over his head and a Chevette in the driveway. But then all the auto plants started closing. People were getting evicted and leaving town. Schools were shutting down. Homes were falling empty and becoming increasingly decrepit. Then the crack epidemic came through and finished it off.

Through it all, there was a feeling of powerlessness, of learned helplessness. People didn't know how to do anything because there was always the expectation that GM would do it for them. When GM collapsed, there was no social infrastructure in place to pick up and carry on without it. The town wasn't capable of starting over on its own. The only thing people could do was rail at the company for taking the jobs away and then sit and wait for the company to bring the jobs back, which of course it never did. So growing up where I did with the family I had, I learned all the wrong lessons about money. I never learned to have control over money, only to let money have control over me.

Learning all the wrong lessons about money started with learning all the wrong lessons about work. On top of working at GM, my dad always used to spend his Saturdays doing handyman jobs in different people's homes—and by "different people" I mean women. Attractive ones, usually. I never knew for sure what was up, but I had my suspicions. He'd always bring Marcelle and me along to help him, too. He'd barge in our room at 5:00 a.m. and turn on the lights, saying, "Let's go! The early bird gets the worm. Let's go! Today we going to work!" It was that military thing he had.

He'd drag us to these ladies' houses and introduce us and say, "These are my sons. They're going to be helping out today." Sometimes he'd make us sit there for hours while he worked under some kitchen sink, passing him wrenches and screwdrivers, watching our Saturday disappear, and hating our lives. Other times he'd bring us there and tell us to mow the lawn, if it was summer, or shovel the driveway, if it was winter. Then he'd leave us there to go off and do God knows what. We'd do the yard, sometimes two or three yards. Then we'd sit and wait hours and hours, often until the sun went down, for him to come back and pick us up. And he never paid us. The women and the families we worked for paid any money to Big Terry, and he kept it, so we'd work all day for nothing. If we asked him about getting paid, he'd say, "I'm teaching you what it's all about. I'm showing you how it is." As far as Big Terry was concerned, not getting paid was part of our lesson.

Once we were a bit older, Marcelle and I started going out and finding our own odd jobs, getting paid a few dollars here and there to mow lawns and shovel snow. My dad, knowing this, always used to come and stand in the doorway to our room and say, "You guys got any money?"

We couldn't lie to him, so we'd say, "Uhhhhh . . . yeah."

"Okay," he'd say. "Lemme see it. Don't worry, I'll give it back."

So we would give him everything we'd saved, and then we'd never see it again. Marcelle was a meticulous saver. At one point, he'd saved up almost $400 under his mattress, which in those days was a crazy amount of money. Then one night my father walked in and snatched it, and my brother never saw that money again.

I learned that lesson quickly: if you get it, spend it. Anytime I had five bucks, I was going to McDonald's or buying some comic books, always making sure I got what I wanted before he could take it. That way, whenever he came around and stood in my doorway asking for money, I could tell him the truth. "I spent it." Then, thinking I was the smart one, I'd watch Marcelle reach under his mattress and fork over whatever he'd scraped together that week.

As a result, I never learned how to work for money, and I never learned how to save money. I even grew to hate the whole idea of "work." All through high school my friends were getting their minimum-wage jobs at the mall or wherever, and I never did. I never wanted to work because it was something I was penalized for instead of being rewarded for. My attitude was "What's the point? Why should I get a job if my dad is going to come along and take the money?"

Of course, I "worked" at my art and "worked" at sports. I threw myself into those things and gave them 110 percent, but those endeavors had no relationship to money. Nobody was paying me to paint, and "working" as a high school athlete in the hopes of going pro means putting your body through grueling punishment day after day in exchange for a less than 1 percent chance that it might pay off one day eight years down the line. In other words, it's gambling. It's playing the numbers. It's turning your life into a sweepstakes.

3

HOW COME I AIN'T GETTIN' MINE?

By the time I left home for college, I had no concept of an honest day's work for an honest day's wage. I had no concept of creating value or being fairly compensated for that value. I'd completely adopted my mother's mentality about money, which was that I wasn't going out into the world to work. I was going to hit it big. I was going to "make it," and then the money would somehow magically be there.

Professional athletes aren't successful in the same way a dentist is successful. A dentist makes a good living. Professional athletes win the big door prize and then they're on easy street. At least, that's what I thought at the time, and as an eighteen-year-old kid looking out at life, that's what I wanted. Success wasn't an affordable house and a nice savings account. Success was becoming rich and famous.

It's a terrible attitude to have, but what's truly dangerous about that mentality are the feelings of resentment and entitlement that come along with it. You cling to that sweepstakes mentality, but it doesn't get you anywhere. You sit around mired in poverty, grousing and complaining. Meanwhile, the people around you are putting in the hours and doing the work to get ahead. You see them moving into the nice house and getting the nice car, and it fills you with bitterness. You think, "Huh. They got theirs, how come I ain't gettin' mine?" Which then turns into "Hey, you got some, how come you don't give me some of yours?"

Obviously, luck and good fortune play a part in everyone's success, mine included. But if you believe success is luck and *only* luck, then of course you think it's unfair that other people get lucky and you don't. That's what happened to my mother. The more she suffered in life, the more she looked at those magazine sweepstakes with a sense of entitlement. She *deserved* to win those contests because of the hardship she'd been through.

The worst of it was her attitude toward her own mother. My grandmother was the opposite of my mom and my dad. She worked at her job at AC Spark Plug for forty years. She never made much, but she saved and saved and saved. She was just stacking her money and being smart with it. By the time she retired, she owned her house and her car and didn't have any debts. I can remember my mom being so resentful and entitled about that, too, always going on about how my grandmother needed to be doing more for us.

I picked up that same sense of entitlement. When I went away to college at Western Michigan, I expected my grandmother to buy me a car. I not only felt like she ought to do it, I was angry at her that she didn't do it, as if I were owed the money this old woman had worked hard for all her life. I didn't even offer to work for half of it or get a job to pay for my gas, nothing. I thought, "She got some, how come I can't get some?" I had that attitude, 100 percent, and as time went on, it only got worse.

Sophomore year, once I made good on my promise and earned a scholarship by making the team, I was certain I was on my way to the NFL. My attitude was that I was the guy in our family who was going to become a star and achieve greatness for all of us. Now I really *was* my mother's sweepstakes. I knew it, and I acted like it. I felt I was entitled to special treatment within my family, which I'm not proud to admit.

That summer I had started working, at least. The school's athletic boosters and alumni would hook players up with jobs, and I got one at a refrigeration company, Stafford-Smith, owned by one of my teammates' fathers. I was a human forklift, hauling refrigeration units to the top floors of buildings. Because I was working, I decided I needed and deserved a car, and I wanted my parents to help pay for it, which they couldn't do; even though I had an art scholarship to cover part of my tuition, they had gone heavily into debt to cover the rest. So I went to my grandmother and said, "I went and got a scholarship, and now I need you to help me get a car." She asked if I was going to pay her back, and I told her I would, out of the money I was making at Stafford-Smith. She agreed to pitch in with a down payment on a Chevy Nova, and I agreed to pay her back and take over the car note once my scholarship came in. Which I never did. I let my grandmother eat the down payment, and I stuck my parents with paying the installments—and I was so arrogant I actually told myself they should feel lucky for the opportunity to be helping me. I was getting the hell out of Flint and going to the NFL, and I was letting them ride along, so they should be grateful.

And what did I do with my money from the refrigeration company? I wish I could remember. Mostly new shoes and new clothes.

Once I met Rebecca, I spent it on taking her out for dinners we both knew I couldn't afford.

"Where'd you get the money for this?" she'd ask, looking at the prices on the menu.

"I just got my check."

"Did you pay your rent?"

"It'll be all right."

Of course, it wasn't all right, because I wasn't paying my rent. At the time I was living off campus with a roommate. I ended up being short several months in a row and, thanks to me, we both had to sneak out in the middle of the night. I feel horrible about it to this day, but back then I didn't take responsibility for myself or my actions. I thought ignoring a situation was the same as fixing it.

After a short turn back to the dorms, I eventually convinced Rebecca that we should share her apartment together even though we weren't married. Plus, with my having a car, if we pooled our resources, we could live better. It made a kind of pragmatic sense if you ignored the flashing red neon sign declaring what a disaster I was, financially and otherwise. So she let me move in.

Rebecca later told me that she saw the flashing red neon sign from the beginning, but she let herself ignore it because she was swept up in the romance of dating. The truth is Rebecca was always industrious, always frugal. She was a single mom on food stamps and welfare, living in a subsidized apartment, trying to get by on the little money she was making at the salon. When she played piano at church, she had to get paid under the table so the government wouldn't see that money and reduce her housing subsidy. Her whole life was about protecting Naomi and doing what was right for her, and I seriously doubt she would have married me if I'd been honest with her about my situation.

In the beginning, we were so broke I was scared that if I ate at home, she and Naomi would run out of food, so I started I sneaking back into my old dormitory to eat, sometimes twice a day. The head of the kitchen was this older white guy who knew I was struggling, and he was kind enough to wave me through the line without paying. He snuck me in so many times he started to get afraid that he would get in trouble, so even that had its limits. There were days I'd be starving and late for practice and I'd go to sneak in and he'd have to stop me. "Sorry, Terry," he'd say. "I can't do it today."

It killed me, but I understood. And while I was always grateful to him, as a person, I can't say that I was grateful in general. I wasn't humbled by my need for an old man's charity. In my mind, I wasn't breaking the rules to make up for my own lack of responsibility with money. I was taking what I needed to take because I was a superstar in waiting and life wasn't giving me what I deserved. Imagine being so broke you have to sneak into a cafeteria to steal food, yet thinking you're so important it's something you're entitled to. It's sad to think I was ever that young and arrogant, but I was.

Rebecca and I got married on July 29, 1989. We couldn't afford a big party, but everybody we knew chipped in and did as much as they could. Instead of a big reception, our wedding was basically a big potluck dinner. In lieu of an actual honeymoon, we had a room for the night at a local bed-and-breakfast. But the joy and happiness I felt that night more than made up for the lack of glitz and glamour. Unfortunately, as the reality of our financial situation set in, it was hard to keep that attitude up.

Foolishly, I'd gotten married with the feeling that stability and normalcy would magically come along with it. Of course, that didn't happen. We were still broke. Instead of developing a serious work ethic to deal with the problem, I kept coming up with schemes and plans that I'd never follow through on. At one point I got it in my mind that I was going to make and sell airbrushed T-shirts. So I took the bit of money we had and bought an airbrush pen and a bunch of ink. Rebecca greeted this notion with a skeptical side-eye. "Are you really going to do this?" she asked. "Because if you buy this equipment, you'd better do it." Of course, I didn't. I was always starting things like that, saying I was going to do them and then never following through.

Then the credit card bills came due. Credit cards were another big problem in my family. When Visa and Mastercard first started giving them out to just about anybody, my aunt was the first to get one. She would take us all to Red Lobster, and it would be a windfall we couldn't believe. Like, "Wait a minute, you mean you give them the card and they give you the food? *What?*" That's how we looked at it. Magic card, magic money. If you could get it on credit, just get it, because everybody else got it, too.

When I got to Western Michigan, the credit card companies were handing out accounts like candy. Working people with jobs couldn't get them, but if you were an unemployed student? "Here, have all you want." And I had them all: American Express, Visa, Mastercard, Discover, even a Sears card. I maxed them all out almost immediately, and by the time Rebecca and I got married, they had all been cut off. I owed thousands of dollars in high-interest debt, something I never told Rebecca before she let me put a ring on her finger. I couldn't even make the minimum payments anymore. One day the repo men came and took the TV back. From then on, we had creditors calling the house looking for me constantly. Probably the lowest moment came when there was a knock on the door, and our upstairs neighbor was standing there looking sheepish.

"Hey, man," he said. "Look, uh . . . Visa is on the line at my house. They're looking for you."

"Oh. I'm sorry, man," I said. "I'll handle it."

But I didn't handle it, and I wasn't sorry. I was angry. I was like all the people back in Flint who'd been taken care of by GM their whole lives, standing around helpless and wondering, "When is GM going to fix this for us?" I'd created my own mess by not working, by maxing out my cards, but I was just sitting around, waiting for someone else to take care of it for me. And whenever Rebecca looked to me to come up with a solution, all I could offer her was my sweepstakes coupon. "We're gonna go pro, baby," I'd say. "And as soon as I go pro, all of these bills are going to be paid. So don't even worry."

"Okay, okay," she said, but she didn't ever sound convinced, and in the meantime the calls kept coming. The stress was of it was unbearable, so I dodged them as much as I could, but one day I was at home trying to study, and I ended up on the phone with a guy from a collection agency. He started getting short with me, and I snapped.

"You know what, man," I said, "In a minute I'm going to be in the NFL, and you are still going to be sitting in your cubicle making what? Eight dollars an hour? Maybe? If that?"

Of course, I'd never made eight dollars an hour doing anything, yet there I was knocking the guy who did. I didn't stop there. "I'm going to be rich," I said. "And you're still going to be working there, calling people, begging for your little money."

Finally, Rebecca grabbed the phone out of my hand and hung it up. A minute later, the phone rang again. It was the same guy. I picked up, fighting mad, ready to get back into it, but then he caught me off guard. "Sir," he said, "you know what, I apologize. Just pay us when you can." And then he hung up.

For a minute I felt good. I even puffed my chest out a bit. My rant had worked. Getting angry had worked. But the relief was momentary. Pretty soon the bills were piling up and the stress came back and, after a brief interruption, the collection calls started coming again. Some days the phone would ring and ring and ring, Naomi would cry and cry and cry, and Rebecca would give me a look, like she was wondering what she had gotten herself into.

4

BETTER THAN GOLD

Making it to the NFL wasn't quite the sweepstakes I imagined it would be. One year after leaving professional football, I was broke. And by "broke" I mean "digging in the couch cushions for change to buy gas" broke. After my last regular season with the Eagles, we moved out to LA and were living in a tiny extended-stay hotel in Burbank. We didn't know a soul. Naomi was ten, Azi was eight, Rebecca was pregnant, and I was a fool. I was still expecting to "hit it big," only in Hollywood instead of football. Compounding that terrible attitude, I now had all the arrogance and entitlement of a professional athlete who expected opportunities to be handed to him. I was concerned about my ego, how I looked, how people saw me. I was "Terry Crews," I'd played in the NFL. I was too proud, and too arrogant, to look for a job. I was just using my pro football connections to try to get meetings and waiting for Hollywood to open its doors to me.

The NFL was supposed to be my golden ticket. The reality was anything but. When I signed with the Los Angeles Rams coming out of Western Michigan, I got paid $75,000. At the time it felt like all the money in the world, but NFL contracts are game to game. There's no guaranteed salary. Since I didn't play a single game my first year, I had to make that seventy-five grand last the whole year. I hadn't learned anything about financial discipline. I was still managing all my credit card debt, and because I never stopped believing my big payday was right around the corner, I kept indulging in all the clothes and nice meals I thought I was entitled to. It was all about feeling good and avoiding pain; if I felt stressed or unhappy, my solution was to go buy something, including a brand-new Nissan Pathfinder we couldn't afford.

The Rams cut me after two seasons, and with no money and nowhere else to go, we moved back in with my parents in Flint. There I was: out washing my brand-new SUV in the driveway while my wife and kids had to share a roof with my dysfunctional parents. Then, I couldn't even keep the Pathfinder in the driveway anymore. I had to start parking it at my grandmother's because the repo man was looking for it. Meanwhile, all the money I'd spent on the car could have gone to put my wife and kids in a real home. I cringe when I think about it now. The humiliation alone should have been enough to make me change my ways, but it didn't.

The rest of my NFL career went pretty much the same. I was a journeyman player, always good enough to get signed by and train with a new team, but never good enough to be one of the greats or even a serious player. I never made more than the absolute minimum a player could legally be paid. Not long after we landed back in Flint I got picked up by the Green Bay Packers. They cut me after training camp. Then the Chargers picked me up, and I flew to San Diego on a moment's notice to make the start of training camp while Rebecca followed me in the car, driving two kids cross-country by herself. When I showed up at practice in San Diego, the repo man was waiting for me in the parking lot, looking for the Pathfinder; these guys were on me coast to coast. Luckily, I managed to tap-dance my way through, explaining that I'd just been signed by the team, and they let me keep the car and start making the payments again.

We were still holding on to the bottom rung of the ladder, but barely. There were times Rebecca would break down crying from the stress. I'd made so many empty promises to her out of my sense of entitlement. I'd gotten us into so many problems with money. I'd kept saying things were going to get better, but they'd only gotten worse. San Diego offered us a brief respite. We managed to keep our heads above water for that year, but then I got cut again.

It was the third team that had let me go in as many years, a tremendous blow. Even Rebecca, whose faith in me had never wavered, was starting to have her doubts.

"You know, honey," she said, "maybe you're not that good."

I felt that. It *hurt*. It was one of those rock-bottom moments that took me right back to the trauma of my childhood. Because if I wasn't worthy of the NFL, then I was worthless. We stumbled through the rest of that year thanks to some money I made painting portraits of some of my teammates. Then it was back on the road: a year with the World League in Germany, a year in DC, and finally a year with the Eagles in Philadelphia and an aborted training camp in San Francisco with the 49ers. Every year would start off the same, me full of hubris and pride that this was going to finally be the big break. Every year would end the same, too, with Rebecca stressed out and crying at the end of each month trying to cover the rent and the bills and keep the kids in school clothes.

It had been obvious since San Diego that things weren't working out, but my stubbornness and my pride kept me from seeing the truth. When we moved to LA with nothing and landed in our little extended-stay hotel, Rebecca kept saying, "You need a job." I kept saying, "Hey, I'm still trying to make this thing happen. I'm a football player and a filmmaker and artist. What will it look like with me working at McDonald's?"

"But Terry," she'd plead, "you need a *job*. We don't have *anything*."

My pride still wouldn't let me do it. I was pawning everything I could put my hands on instead. I hocked Rebecca's wedding ring, my watch. It was a bad time. The only reason we made it through was my friend Ken Harvey.

Ken Harvey and I had played together in DC. He was one of the stars of the team, and also one of the first NFL linebackers to make big money. The first time I ever shared a practice field with him, I hit him so hard he started bleeding—he has a scar on his neck from it to this day—and in the dog-eat-dog, Marlboro Man world of professional football, Ken was one of my few true friends. He'd invite me over to his house to shoot pool or hang out and talk. He liked to write, and he admired my paintings, so we bonded over that. Those nights were such a relief after what I'd seen earlier in my NFL career, with the guns and the drugs and the strip clubs. I still had my trusty old Pathfinder, and when it broke down, Ken let me borrow his Mercedes-Benz. Now that's a friend.

After we moved out to LA, Ken was my lifeline. At the time, a lot of financial advisers were telling people to invest in gold bullion as a hedge against inflation, and Ken had become a bit of a gold bug, accumulating a big pile of gold coins. He wanted to help me make it in Hollywood, but he couldn't mail me checks without his wife knowing about it. So every few weeks he'd send me one of his coins. "Each coin is an ounce," he said, "If you get into any money trouble, take the coin to a jeweler. Whatever the price of gold is that day, they'll give you that much." They usually cashed in for around $300.

He probably sent me fifteen or so over the course of our first year in LA. It got to the point where I was basically a dependent, all because I was too proud to go get a damn job. When that first year was up, I finally hit rock bottom: I hocked my car. Which in LA is suicide. You can't live—you can barely even function—without a car. Pretty soon, the money from hocking the car was gone, too, at which point I was completely screwed.

I called Ken. "Dude, I need some help," I said. "Can you send me just a little bit?"

"Terry," he said, taking a deep breath, "I can't do it."

In all the years we'd been friends, it was the first time he'd ever said no. I was stunned. I didn't know what to say. It was that horrible moment of shame where I realized I'd overstepped.

"Why not?" I asked.

"Hey, man, it's just . . . it's enough," he said. "I've given you all of the money I can. The reason I gave you the coins was because my wife would have felt uncomfortable with me writing checks. But it's not right to keep doing this to her. This is her money, too. I can't give you any more."

"Hey, I understand," I said. "No problem. I'll talk to you later."

But what I said was not how I felt. In that moment, instead of being grateful for everything he'd done for me, I got mad. I have rarely been angrier at any human being than I was at that moment. I said to myself, "Fuck him! He's supposed to be a friend, and he won't even help me at the time I need it the most?! Fuck Ken Harvey!"

It was so violent, I felt like I might actually kill him. The feeling lingered for only a few minutes, and then all of a sudden I realized, "Wait a minute. Why am I mad at the only person who's been trying to help me in the first place?"

And the reason I was so angry was that I'd become entitled. It was that same mentality I'd had growing up: "He got some, how come I can't get some?" It was the same learned helplessness that had plagued so many others in Flint. Ken had become my GM. I was a grown man, but I was expecting him to take care of me. I'd become so dependent on that help that I hadn't learned how to do for myself.

At 5:00 a.m. the next day I went over to a place called Labor Ready, which I knew about because I'd driven by it a few times. It was an employment agency where you could show up and wait and get assigned to work an eight-hour gig somewhere. It was a more organized version of those guys who stand around outside Home Depot waiting for work crews to come by in pickups and say, "I need five workers," and then they all run and jump in the truck.

The vibe at Labor Ready was basically like a halfway house. Many of the workers had just come out of prison. They were in rough shape. There were homeless people and drug addicts, too, dirty and scratching themselves. That's when the realization hit me hard: I was no better than them.

The agency sent me to a place in the Valley, some factory called White Cap, where I was handed a broom to start sweeping. The moment I took it in my hand, I thought I was going to die. I thought I was going to throw up. I could not believe how far my life had come down, from the NFL to *this*. I had tears in my eyes when I started sweeping. The voice in my head kept saying, "You suck. You failed. You're nothing. Here you were telling everybody that you were going to be this big shot. Now look at you. You're going to do this for the rest of your life."

That moment broke me—in all the good ways. It brought me to my knees. It humbled me. It forced me to look myself in the mirror and swallow my pride. It forced me to do the thing that I was most scared of in life: I had to admit that I'd been wrong. Wrong about everything, but especially about money. I wasn't entitled to it. I hadn't ever earned it. There was no big sweepstakes victory waiting right around the corner.

I swept that floor for eight hours. The first hour was pure misery, but as I swept, this magical feeling came over me: I was actually *doing* something about my situation. I was working. For the first time in my life. Don't get me wrong, I busted my ass in the NFL. I killed myself out on that field. But I was never in control of what I was doing. In the NFL, the team signs you or doesn't sign you. The team trades you or drops you. All you do is wait for the phone to ring so someone can tell you what to do. I'd been stuck in that mentality, waiting for someone else to help me or tell me what to do or just do everything for me. But the moment I started sweeping, I wasn't waiting for someone to call anymore. I wasn't wondering when some big break was going to come my way. For the first time in my life, I was *working*.

It felt so good. I swept every inch of that damn floor. I was getting in the corners, under the boxes. The busier I got, the less I thought about my troubles. I started thinking about the money I was going to get at the end of the day and the smile on Rebecca's face when I brought it home. I worked the whole eight hours, went back to Labor Ready, and presented my slip to folks working there. My wage was eight dollars an hour, which came to a total of sixty-four dollars, which, after taxes, came to forty-eight dollars. They'd cash it for you right there, so when I left, I had forty-eight dollars in my hand. I put twenty in the gas tank, went home, gave twenty to Rebecca, and I had eight in my pocket. It wasn't much, but it was eight dollars that I hadn't had the day before.

I knew from that moment on that I would never be broke again. Because I knew there was no job too low that I wouldn't do it to support my family. To me it was like an epiphany, a revelation. Of course, when I shared all this with Rebecca, she was like, "I know. I've been telling you this for years."

That same night I picked up the phone and called Ken Harvey, to apologize for overstepping, to thank him for his generosity and for cutting me off. Because his cutting me off, more than his generosity, was what saved me. Ken Harvey telling me no was the best thing that ever happened to me. To this day I call it my Ken Harvey Wake-Up Moment. It was a rebirth, a giant leap forward.

After sweeping floors for a week, I bounced over to a temp agency that sent me to the Veterans Administration, where I had to reorganize an archive of files that had fallen over in an earthquake. It was mind numbing, literally just me in a cubicle for eight hours a day, re-alphabetizing massive stacks of paperwork. But day after day, I tackled it the same way I tackled those factory floors. It was another good lesson: life is full of work you don't want to do, so when you're faced with work you don't want to do, use it as an opportunity to learn how to work faster and more efficiently, so you can get past the thing you don't want to be doing—a mentality that would serve me well in Hollywood in the years to come.

While I was temping in the file room, I started bouncing at bars and clubs on the side. Doing that, I met a former cop who liked my upbeat attitude, which is something you don't see in a lot of bouncers. This cop introduced me to a company called Cast Security that did security for big movie sets. I went in and they hired me right away and, finally, there it was: My sweepstakes coupon. My big break.

Because that's how life actually works. Luck doesn't fall on you from the sky. You can't just name it and claim it. Yes, it's luck, and you don't control when or where it happens—or if it's good luck or bad—but it comes only if you're working for it. It comes as the fruit of what you're putting out into the universe. For a long time, the only vibe I was giving off was arrogance, selfishness, and entitlement, and nothing came my way. After my experience at Labor Ready, I was giving off only exuberance and enthusiasm and dedication, no matter how menial the task. People noticed.

With Cast Security, I started working on movie sets, Jim Carrey's *Man on the Moon*, Arnold Schwarzenegger's *End of Days*. I didn't look like your average movie set security guard. I would iron my shirts, stand at attention. I would be pleasant and upbeat all day, and I wasn't faking it. As far as I was concerned, I was in the movie business. Doing any job on a film set, to me, was like paid film school. I decided to make every day a learning experience, to make good use of every single moment of every single shift. There were days when I worked twelve hours straight. Since I didn't have time to go to the gym, I'd jog in place for an hour, and that was my day's workout. If there was a light pole without many people around, I'd jump on it and do pull-ups, then drop on the ground and do push-ups, too.

I didn't let my brain atrophy, either. I went to the library and filled up a gym bag with books on the entertainment industry. When no one was looking, I read book after book after book. I even wrote scripts standing up sometimes. I spent every day filled with joy from the privilege of being at this job.

One afternoon, while working on *End of Days*, Arnold Schwarzenegger's makeup artist, a guy named Jeff Dawn, walked by me and said, "Dude, are you a security guard?"

"Yes, I am, sir."

"You should be in there on the set. You need to be in the movies. You've got a great look."

I thought he was hitting on me. "Thank you, sir," I said.

"No, man. I'm *telling* you. You belong in front of a camera."

I shrugged it off. I'd only ever wanted to work in the movie business, not be in movies themselves. Then the same thing happened on a couple of other sets, so I asked Rebecca, "Do you think I should try this acting thing? People keep telling me I should."

"It can't hurt," she said. "We've got nothing else. Go for it."

So I went for it. A guy I knew through Cast Security heard about auditions for a new reality show, a modern-day gladiator competition called *Battle Dome*. I went in, I auditioned, and I got it.

A year later I got my first major acting job in Schwarzenegger's next movie, *The 6th Day*. When I walked into the makeup trailer, Jeff Dawn was there, and he said, "Hmm, you look familiar . . ."

"I know," I said. "A year ago I was working as a security guard on *End of Days* and you told me I should be in the business. And here I am."

"Oh my God!" he exclaimed. "I remember you. Standing outside the place! And now you're here on this movie. I'm making people rich, I knew it! I knew it!"

And that's when stuff started happening. From that moment came *Training Day. Friday after Next. White Chicks. The Longest Yard. Idiocracy.* It all started with a broom and me crying my eyes out sweeping up a factory floor. That was the moment that saved my life, because that was the first moment in my life when I learned how to work and provide for myself and my family.

5

A VIRTUOUS CYCLE

After my stint at Labor Ready, I'd finally fixed my relationship with work, and we were finally making regular, decent money. Unfortunately, I still hadn't fixed my relationship with money. I'd fixed my attitude about getting the money, but I hadn't fixed my attitude about keeping the money. I was still going through it as fast as I could make it.

When *Everybody Hates Chris* got picked up for air in 2005, I was no longer just making decent money. We had real money coming in for the first time in our lives: a regular, steady stream of income where you actually got to sit and make choices about what kind of life you wanted. For starters, we upgraded our lives accordingly. We rented a five-bedroom house in a gated community in Altadena. It was the biggest house we'd ever lived in, palatial compared with anywhere else we'd ever stayed. But I wasn't content to have the nice house in the good neighborhood. I picked up all those trappings of fame people make you feel like you're supposed to have, like a publicist. I didn't need a publicist. Brad Pitt needs a publicist. I wasn't a movie star; I was an ensemble player on a well-liked and modestly successful sitcom. But I felt I needed to project an image that wasn't real. I got caught up in wanting all the Hollywood status symbols. I wanted the nice car, the nice clothes. One time I even wore sunglasses indoors at a party.

Yeah, I was that guy.

My ego was the single biggest line item in our monthly budget, and the cars and the clothes were the least of it. Long before I started acting, my dream had been to be behind the scenes, making and producing movies. I'd always fancied myself as being from the Do-It-Yourself Spike Lee–Michael Moore school of filmmaking. I'd seen what they'd done with *She's Gotta Have It* and *Roger and Me*. They'd spent their own money and made their movies, and then success had followed.

During my NFL days, in 1995, a former teammate and I began filming a movie he'd written called *Young Boys Inc*. He was the director and I decided to be the producer. I put my own money into it, and we even filmed a few scenes on the mean streets of Detroit. But we never finished. We got threatened by some of the actual Young Boys, who wanted tell us how the movie should go. Then we ran out of money. I tried to generate some heat to raise the money to finish it. I threw a big fundraiser with a bunch of my teammates in DC and spent nearly $20,000 on an event to impress them, hoping they'd invest in the movie. They ate, drank, and left. I didn't earn a single cent back on the whole endeavor.

I was doing the same thing during *Everybody Hates Chris*. I had ideas for films I wanted to make. Now that I was in with the Chris Rocks and Adam Sandlers of the business, I thought I had the connections to do something. I probably spent over $100,000 trying to get different projects off the ground. None of them ever worked.

I didn't even begin to understand the real problem until much later on: I wasn't really spending money on clothes and cars and passion projects. I was spending money in a futile effort to be happy. I was so incapable of sitting with and dealing with my own unhappiness that I would do anything to lift myself out of it. Every time I was sad, I needed to get happy, so I spent money to get that dopamine hit I needed. I made risky, ridiculous, impulsive decisions, all because I was trying to improve my state of mind or pump up my ego.

Meanwhile, all this money was flying out the door. I wasn't paying attention to my taxes, and I ran up quite a tab with Uncle Sam. I kept pushing it off and pushing it off, saying to myself, "The next gig is going to pay it off." That was my mindset. But the debt kept getting bigger and bigger. By the time I finally faced the music and started paying it down, it had ballooned to about six hundred grand.

Around 2011, when I finally turned to confront the debt monster I'd created, I did what I always did when dealing with my problems: I picked up a book. Lots of them, actually. I read everything about personal financial planning and management I could put my hands on, but the book that really made a difference for me was called *The Richest Man in Babylon*, by George S. Clason. It had all the usual advice about living within your means and not investing in enterprises you don't fully understand, but the one piece of advice from this book that resonated with me was how important it is to give to charity—and not just to give to charity, but to do what the Bible says and tithe 10 percent of your income to charity. Every year. No matter how much or how little you make. The minute I read that, something clicked. It made perfect sense. From the beginning of our marriage, the practice of tithing was another thing Rebecca had always requested I do, right along with get a job. As with most things, she'd been right all along, and I was the one late to the party.

The biblical reason for tithing 10 percent of your income is to create a virtuous circle. It's karma. Reaping what you sow. Paying it back by paying it forward. Whatever you want to call it. The universe gives to you only what you give back to the universe. Put goodness and kindness into the world, and goodness and kindness will return to you. And that's true. I 100 percent believe that to be true. But the minute I read about tithing in this book, I intuitively knew there was a far more practical, tangible reason for tithing as well.

Once I started tithing, I realized it was like hitting the gym. For the seven years I was in the NFL, I stayed in incredible shape, because it was my job to stay in shape. The minute I left the league and we moved to LA, all that discipline went out the window. I got *fat*. I was so focused on making something happen in movies that I stopped going to the gym. I was living on burgers and fast food. I woke up one morning and realized I'd put on forty pounds like it was nothing. I was tired all the time, lethargic, sluggish, and I was in complete denial about it, too, schlubbing around the house in nothing but baggy T-shirts and sweatpants to avoid looking at the problem.

Then one morning Rebecca came up behind me at the bathroom sink and pinched my back fat.

"What did you just do?" I said, tensing up.

"What?" she said. "You got a little thing here, that's all."

Then she pinched it again.

"Stop," I said. "Stop, stop."

"Why? It's cute. It's all right, honey. I love you. It doesn't matter to me."

But it *did* matter to me. That was all it took to send me back to the gym. I found enough money in the couch cushions to pay for a gym membership, and I started working out again. As I walked into the locker room for the first time, I thought about something the pastor at our church in San Diego had once said to me, that if you force yourself to do something for twenty-one days, it will become a habit, which means no matter how bad your circumstance is, you can change your life in twenty-one days. The hard part is recognizing that you need to change.

Getting back to working out was brutal. I was only a year out from being a professional athlete, and I could barely go five minutes on the recumbent bike. The first few times I went, I just got on that bike, read a magazine, and went home. But no matter how bad it felt, or how down I got, I made myself go back every day, and, sure enough, within twenty-one days, I was doing full workouts again. The weight came off. My mood improved. My mind was clearer. Same as sweeping those floors, the act of doing something about my situation gave me an incredible boost of self-esteem.

We always tell ourselves we don't have time to spend an hour exercising every day. We're too busy with work and with family. But the thing about the hour of exercise is that it makes you feel so much better that the other twenty-three hours of the day become that much more productive. Giving up that hour of time actually gets you more time, because it gives you better use of your time. You sleep better. You work more efficiently. You eat better, too, and not because you're forcing yourself on some diet you hate, but because your body doesn't want that unhealthy food anymore. More than anything, it forces you to manage your time to make sure you have that hour for the gym, and that fact alone ensures that you're paying attention to your days and making the most of every moment.

Tithing 10 percent of your income is like that hour at the gym. It's a way of imposing discipline on yourself. It's giving something up to get more in return. Because that's how the world operates. That's how *everything* operates. It's a basic, universal principle. There is no free lunch. You never get something for nothing. The sweepstakes and the lotteries are BS. Tithing is the diametric opposite of the sweepstakes mentality I'd grown up with. In order to receive, you first have to give. It's not "They got theirs, how come I ain't getting mine?" It's "Let me give to them so that I get mine in return."

I went straight to my business manager and said, "I want to start tithing ten percent of everything I make." Now, mind you, I was making good money in TV, but I still owed hundreds of thousands of dollars to the IRS. I had a wife and five kids and college tuition to pay for. My business manager looked at me like I was crazy.

"Terry," he said. "You can't give up ten percent, you'll go broke."

"I don't care," I said. "I'll adjust. But I need to do this."

"Terry, you can't afford to do this."

"I can't afford *not* to do it."

I told his firm to do it, but that didn't get it done. A year later, when Rebecca accidentally got cc'd on an email, we found out they'd been telling us that they were paying the tithes, but they hadn't actually done it. They'd held on to my money after I told them to give it away—because they thought I was nuts!

So I fired them.

I decided to take over our finances myself, and that was a whirlwind. I bought budgeting books, a bunch of different money-tracking apps and worksheets. I even hired an accountant to come in to work for me directly and help me do our spreadsheets.

Just like the first five minutes I spent on that recumbent bike, the first year of tithing was brutal. It was maybe one of the most painful things I've ever done. But I swallowed that pain, and it gave me a new perspective. I started budgeting, watching where every dollar came in and how every dollar went out, *for real*. I spent a week carrying around a notebook and forced myself to write down every cent I spent, every time I spent it. I realized how quickly the money was going. I wrote down every transaction: $10 for this, $20 for that, and the next thing I knew $300 was gone. I was shocked.

From then on, I cut all the unnecessary spending. I paid all my bills on time, I watched every penny. Once I had everything the way I wanted it, I brought in new financial managers. Initially, they butted heads with me over the tithing, too. They also thought it was crazy. But I sat down with them and said, "Guys, I don't care if I go broke. I want ten percent going to my church off the gross. I'll accept full responsibility for whatever happens."

They shrugged and agreed to do it, and not only did our spending and money management stay on track, not long after that, I started to get one major opportunity after the other: a new Old Spice campaign, *The Expendables 2*, *Brooklyn Nine-Nine*, *Who Wants to Be a Millionaire*, *World's Funniest Fails*, a Toyota Super Bowl commercial. I started seeing offers that were double and triple what I'd seen before. It was the most profitable time we'd ever seen in our lives, and we've never looked back. Rebecca had been telling me to do this our whole marriage, and when she saw how committed I was to it, she started to see every new opportunity as the fruit of our new tithing habit.

Tithing helped me save money and earn more money. It also set me free from worry. It gave me a peace of mind I'd never had before. I'd had bill collectors and creditors and the IRS hanging over me since college. The stress of that had been like a jackhammer in my head, loud and incessant. Once it was gone, the level of Zen-like peace I achieved was like nothing I'd ever felt. Once I experienced that, there was no going back.

I've lived that way ever since, and today I have zero debt. I'm free. I don't owe anybody anything, the government is paid, and the money in the bank is mine. And I make more money by doing that, because I have a level of comfort that allows me to work better. There is no strain and no stress. I don't have that jackhammer going in my head all the time. Every financial decision I make comes from a position of strength, a position of peace and rightness within myself.

More than anything, tithing completely changed my understanding of what money is. Growing up in the hood, money was *everything*. You didn't have it, so you had to get it. It didn't matter where it came from or how you got it, either: a sweepstakes, playing the numbers, running up a credit card, maybe doing something that wasn't entirely legal. Didn't matter, as long as you got it. Like my dad coming home with the money in his pockets, money was a tangible thing to put your hands on.

But that's wrong, and tithing helped me understand that. Tithing helped me understand that money doesn't really exist. It's a symbol, a representation of value given for value received. When I went into my first shift sweeping floors for Labor Ready, I thought I'd hit rock bottom, but the money I made that day felt better than almost any other dollar I've ever made, because I made it by providing value to my wife and my family. There was a direct correlation between the cash that I was given and the good that it provided.

In the hood, money was all about status. It was about having the biggest gold chain and the Louis Vuitton baggage, the polo with the logo on the front, and the car with the spinning rims that said, "I made it." Throughout my NFL career, that was my whole mentality. I was just about getting that money to buy the nice clothes and the Nissan Pathfinder I couldn't afford. I wanted to show how much I was winning by how much I was spending.

But it's a truly empty way to live. It's even worse if you make all that money doing something that is of no benefit to humanity. Wall Street traders making bank off of gaming the system, casino magnates, pornographers—sure, they might rake it in for a while, but it usually goes bust in the end because they have to keep buying and spending on more and more status symbols to make up for the fact that their lives are so hollow.

For years, part of the reason I was unable to see the correlation between money and value was that I didn't value myself. Knowing that I was lying to my wife about my infidelity and my addiction, I discounted what I was worth, all the time. Just feeling that way, even subconsciously, made me accept less in all my deals. Not knowing the truth, Rebecca didn't understand. She was always saying, "Terry, you deserve more. Why are you taking less?" And I would say, "Well, this is all I can get, and I've gotta be appreciative of it."

Once I became more out in the open and transparent and vulnerable and honest, I could feel better about demanding more because I felt my own value had increased. Negotiating my latest deal with NBC for *America's Got Talent*, I knew that I'd added value to the show, and I knew that was worth something. So I stood my ground and asked for it—and I got it.

You don't work for money. You work for appreciation. You work to create value and to be valued. What we're seeing at this moment, with millions of people leaving their jobs in the wake of COVID, is telling. People are reevaluating their lives because of this tragedy we've all been through. Businesses can't stay open because they can't find workers. They're begrudgingly raising the wages they're willing to pay, which is a good thing, but at the end of the day, it isn't about the money. It's about being valued in your job and believing your work creates value. At the end of *Do the Right Thing*, Sal balls up money and throws it in Mookie's face. No one wants to get money like that. It's no way to run a business or a country. Because money is only what it symbolizes, and once people understand that, they only want money that's value given for value received.

I always seek to provide value in the entertainment that I create, but in addition to that, tithing makes every dollar I earn valuable no matter what, because 10 percent of every dollar is going to someone in need. When the Bible speaks of giving back, it tells the story of farmers who, when harvesting from their orchards, always leave something on the vine for those who have nothing. If you have ten apples, you pick nine and leave one. That's what I do. Ten percent of every dollar I make goes to pay for a shelter to help a woman like my mom escape a man like my dad. Ten percent of every dollar I make goes to helping a kid like my childhood friend Chris stay off the streets. Ten percent of every dollar I make goes to helping students get the kind of scholarship that would have allowed me to follow my dream of going to art school. Because I tithe, everything I do has value.

When I bring up tithing, people always ask me, "How do you make money by giving money away?" But the fact is that tithing creates a virtuous cycle. Money has to flow like a river. If you dam it up and keep it all to yourself, you've stopped the flow of the river, and eventually it's going to run dry and there's nothing more coming back to you. Meanwhile, you blow what you've got on fancy cars and clothes to make up for the emptiness in your life, and eventually you're broke. By releasing it and letting it flow, you've created a bigger waterway, and more money is going to come back your way. And that sounds very Pollyanna and kumbaya. But it's the only way society works.

Just as I learned that the best thing to do with my strength as a man was to put it in service of other people, the same thing is true of money. The best way to become successful is to serve people. The more people you serve, the more valued you are. The more valued you are, the more you receive, which can come in the form of more money, or it can come in the form of other intangibles that are worth more than money, like happiness, respect, and a sense of purpose. Work becomes its own blessing. So now, the question I ask myself every morning is not "How do I make more money?" The question I ask myself is "How do I increase my value?"

IV

AGENCY

1

THE AUX CORD

I was riding in the car one afternoon with my son. He said he wanted to listen to some music, so he pulled out his phone and said, "Hey, give me the aux cord."

"Aux cord?" I thought. "What's he talking about?"

Then I realized he meant the auxiliary input for the stereo. Apparently "aux cord" was what the kids were calling it now. Back in my day, there was no aux cord. You were lucky if you had a cassette deck. There was only the radio, and that dial belonged to one person: the adult who was driving. They chose what everybody listened to. If you didn't like it, tough.

Now, everybody has a device and anybody can jack in. I handed my son the aux cord, and he plugged in his phone and started blasting the latest single from Brockhampton. I liked it, thankfully, because now that's what we were listening to. That's when it kind of hit me: if you're in the car and you've got a long trip ahead of you, you better be careful who you give that aux cord to.

As we drove, I started to think about an experience I'd had a few years earlier working on *Everybody Hates Chris*. There was a guy I worked with on the show. We got along well, and he would come by my dressing room all the time and we'd hang out and talk. Most days he wanted to talk about the problems he was having with his wife. Everything was "she's too this" and "she's upset about that." As you do in those situations, I'd commiserate with him. "Yeah, man. I hear you. My wife does that all the time." At first it was a way to have a laugh and pass the time, but eventually these hangouts turned into gripe sessions about marriage. Fast-forward a couple of months, and I found myself at home, getting irritated by every little thing Rebecca did, even if she wasn't doing anything. I'd just be in a bad mood. That's when I realized, "It's him. It's that guy." I'd given him my aux cord. I'd let him jack right into my mind and influence my thoughts. No marriage is perfect, of course, but this guy and his gripe sessions were slowly but surely making me focus almost entirely on the things about my wife and my marriage that I didn't like, instead of focusing on the positive things that I knew were wonderful. Once I realized what these gripe sessions were doing, I started making myself busy whenever he came by. "Can't talk right now, man! Sorry! Gotta go." Once I did that, right away I started appreciating my marriage again. I was less irritable, and my attitude improved.

It's been said that you are not the voice in your head. You are the person who hears it. We all have those voices, those strange intrusive thoughts that we don't want. Sometimes the voice comes from clear out of nowhere. Sometimes it's bubbling up from somewhere deep in your subconscious. But there's a good chance that the ideas you're hearing are coming from the last person or the loudest person who had your ear. Advertisers know it. Cult leaders know it. Con men know it. Politicians know it. Those types of people are extremely skilled at getting into our heads.

It's tempting to think, "I'm my own person." It's easy to say, "Oh, I'm not going to listen to that." But no matter what you do or where you go in life, other people are always there. No man is an island. We live in a society, in tribes, in families. We need those relationships in some way or another. Some dependencies are easier to deal with. If you have a problem with pornography, you can abstain from pornography. If you have a problem with drugs, you can abstain from drugs. But if you have a problem with food, you still need food. Relationships are the same as food.

The hardest thing in the world is to remain connected to and interdependent with other people, to take and give advice, yet still know your own mind, to hear all the competing voices in your head and know, with certainty, which one is your own. Because somebody's always got your aux cord. It could be an abusive boss or it could be a million Twitter trolls swarming after you. Somebody's always jacked in. Which is why you always have to be cognizant of who that person is and how much power they have over you. Like my son with his iPhone, whoever's got that cord controls what you hear, which means they can set your mood. If they can set your mood, they can influence how you feel. If they can influence how you feel, they can change the way you think. And if they can change the way you think, they can control the way you behave.

2

PLEASER

When you're a child, your parents not only have your aux cord, they *are* your aux cord. For several years, virtually every input you have comes either from them or through them. For me, that typically meant my mom. Big Terry was a domineering presence, but anytime he had my aux cord, I only ever picked up one of two signals: When he was sober, he wouldn't talk. When he was drunk, he would either be crying and rambling or violently screaming. It was static and silence on one hand, bellowing anger on the other. I learned early on to give my aux cord to my dad as rarely as possible.

Trish was different. My mother owned us. We were her property. We did what she said when she said it. But as abusive and controlling and melancholy as my mother could be, when she was in a good mood, she was a joy. I never saw her happier than when she was being entertained. There was a guy named Bill Kennedy on Detroit television back then. He hosted *At the Movies* at one o'clock on WDIV,

Channel 4. They were always classic old Hollywood films. Not a black person anywhere in a single frame, but she loved them. Her favorite show, hands down, was *The Carol Burnett Show*. She *loooooved* Carol Burnett. That was always one of the most enjoyable things that me and my mom would do, piling together on the couch to watch Carol Burnett. My mom would laugh and laugh, her mood would brighten, and the darkness and the violence would go away. Every time.

So I wanted to make her laugh, too.

Like most children of alcoholics and abusers, I was a pleaser. If something would bring peace to the house, I'd do it. What I wanted rarely entered into the equation, because nothing I wanted was as important as keeping things calm. It was always "Make everyone happy. Be a good boy. Don't rock the boat."

With my mother I soon found I could do more than simply pacify her anger. I could create joy. If I could make her laugh, I could pull her out of a dark place—or, better yet, stop her from plunging into one. I could take the signal that was coming in on the aux cord and flip it from negative to positive, like flipping a switch. To this day, if you ask most black guys of my generation who inspired them to get into comedy, nine out of ten will say Richard Pryor. For me it was Carol Burnett. Everything about my love for comedy and entertainment was born out of the experience of watching that show with my mother. On the mornings after Big Terry beat her, she'd be sitting up in bed nursing a black eye or a swollen lip, holding a bag of frozen peas on her face to take down the swelling. I would always go in to try to make her laugh by acting out her favorite Carol Burnett bits, like Mrs. Wiggins or Nora Desmond or Scene Stealing Extras. I can still close my eyes today and see Trish, cracking up with that bag of frozen peas on her face. Just hearing her laugh and seeing her smile told me we'd get through the day, and I'd be okay.

Trish loved to see me dance, too. She was always showing me off.

I started doing the robot when I was five years old. I would be fooling around in the kitchen, popping in time to the beat, and she'd pull me out into the living room where her friends were and say, "Ooh, show everyone that move you were doing." From then on, I was the guy at the family reunion doing the newest dance. My aunt thought I was so good at doing the robot that she'd have me over to kids' birthday parties and coworkers' birthday parties. "Do that robot thang!" she'd say, and I'd do it and they'd all go, "Ohhhhhh!" and I'd be going, "Yes! Approval!" I'd even paint my face and clothes and gloves with silver metallic paint for effect.

I'm that way with my art, too. I started drawing the year Marcelle went to kindergarten. I'd kneel over the blank paper and draw for hours, lost in sketches of monsters and muscled heroes. Whenever I finished a picture and held it up, my mom would beam with pride. It would be a ray of sunshine in the darkness.

Even better, all the girls at school were always going, "Ooh, draw me! Draw me!" Which, for a teenage boy, was the greatest feeling in the world. My good friend Ron Croudy, who's now a successful graphic designer in New York, and I used to do big colorful portraits of all the superstars of the day, like Michael Jordan or Prince. We were known around school, and of course that brought the girls. I must have sketched or painted nearly every girl I liked in school. They would take the print and hold it and go, "Oh my god!" and marvel at how close I got to their likeness. To get that kind of reaction? I was hooked.

I went looking for those same feelings of approval at church. The only person my mom loved more than Carol Burnett was Jesus, and at church I became the poster child for getting involved. Other kids were necking in the bathroom, sneaking off and smoking cigarettes and weed, all kinds of forbidden stuff. I was the opposite of that. I was there for every service, every youth group meeting. I knew it was another way to earn my mother's affection, to make the elders in in our church like me, and to make God like me. Which was all I wanted.

The kids who were misbehaving, they weren't that different from me, actually. When you see poor kids in the hood acting out, a lot of them are trying to find out if anybody gives a damn about them, because their whole lives they've grown up with the feeling that nobody does. They get themselves sent to the principal's office or they get a D on a test just to ask, "Is anyone coming to rescue me? Does anyone care?" So those kids were behaving in a negative way, while I was behaving in what parents would call a "positive" way, but it was all the same unhealthy behavior. It was all driven by "Please look at me. Please notice me. Please care about me."

It's okay, as a kid, to be other directed. You don't know who you are yet, so you look outside of yourself, to parents and peers and mentors. You're looking for cues about what kind of person to be. That's healthy and normal. But I was almost entirely other directed. Compared with the healthier kids from more normal homes, as they were maturing and developing a kind of internal structure to their personalities, I wasn't doing anything of the sort. I lacked any kind of self-guiding rudder or compass to help me chart my own way; it was all about getting the reaction and the feedback I needed from other people in the moment I needed it.

The thing that saved my life and got me out of Flint was that I got lucky. I had two teachers, two mentors, who recognized my potential. They grabbed my aux cord and shouted into it, telling me that I was a good person and a talented person and a person who deserved to believe in himself. One was my art teacher, Mr. Eichelberg, who praised me and pumped me up and paved the way for me to get the scholarship that allowed me to go to Western Michigan. The other was Coach Lee.

By high school I firmly believed, rightly or wrongly, that professional sports and the military were my only chances of escaping Flint. Of the two, I knew that enlisting was the only one that would earn Big Terry's respect. When I began to show interest and promise on the field, he not only didn't encourage it, he actively denigrated it.

Lee Williams was the head coach of the Flint Academy junior varsity football team. For the three years he had me, from seventh through ninth grade, he took an interest in me, becoming the positive father figure I'd never had.

After two years of watching me on the field, in ninth grade, when I was fourteen years old, he said the words that would change my life forever. One day after practice he sat me down. He had this stilted, Army sergeant way of talking. "Terry Crews," he said, "there is no way that you should not be playing football at a Division I school on a Division I scholarship." He would always say my first and last name like that, too. "Terry Crews, you have the ability to do all this. I don't see any athlete in Flint right now that can touch you."

Growing up, I didn't get a lot of compliments. I had never heard anyone say anything like that to me before, and I wouldn't again until I met Mr. Eichelberg in the upper grades. I held on to those words for dear life. Coach Lee believed I should be playing football on a Division I scholarship, and that was what I was going to do.

At the time, my grades were tanking. When I brought home a 1.6 GPA, my parents told me I had to quit playing, which was not an unreasonable position to take. Coach Lee saw the situation from a different angle; he believed keeping me in football, with the incentive of making it to a Division I school, would be the incentive I needed to get my grades up. He came to my house on a Saturday, sat with my parents, and said, "Mrs. and Mr. Crews, I think it would be a big mistake if you do not give Terry this opportunity. This is a way that he'll be able to go to college. He can be a prime athlete. His athletic ability is there, and we're gonna get him there with his grades." My mom wasn't sure, but Coach Lee convinced her. "Mrs. Crews," he said, "let me take care of it." Then he turned to me and said, "I'm putting myself on the line for you. So now you gotta improve, bro. It's up to you."

When he said that, I thought, "If he can do this for me, I can get my grades up for him." I made the honor roll every semester after that.

The irony is that Coach Lee's approval meant so much to me, and I was such a pleaser and approval seeker to my core, that I spent the next decade chasing a dream that wasn't *actually mine*. I gave everything to that game: my blood, my body, and my soul. Then one day years later while I was in the NFL, I was out on the field at practice and I realized, "Wait a minute. I don't actually like football." Because I didn't. I just liked being outside and the camaraderie that came with being a part of a team. The game itself? Never liked it one bit. But Coach Lee's praise meant that much to me. His was the only voice I heard in the darkness, so I followed it.

Coach Lee left Flint Academy not long after he put me on that path. I missed him terribly, but he'd already had an enormous impact on my life. I never had another football coach like him again. My varsity coaches were never supportive. My senior year, I played for a new coach, Coach Thomas. He was the opposite of Coach Lee in every way. Everything with him was negative motivation. He would literally tell you, "You ain't goin' nowhere. You ain't never gonna be nothin'." When I was applying to colleges and trying to get a scholarship, I went to him and asked if I could get some film of me on the field to show to prospective schools. He looked at me and said, "Why?"

His dismissive attitude lit a fire in me. I was like, "Fuck this guy. I'll show him." But that isn't exactly a healthy kind of motivation.

And, either way, I was still being driven not from within, by what I wanted, but from without, by reacting to what others were telling me and doing to me.

In college, my coaches were straight up abusive and racist, and the dynamic didn't change. My only other mentors and friends on campus were a part of Maranatha, the religious cult that had kept me isolated and dependent. Until I met Rebecca, I had no one. I was all alone. And if you're like I was at that point in my life, entirely dependent on other people for any kind of direction or sense of self-worth, to look around and not see a soul? That's a dark, dark moment. Those kinds of moments are the reason people go back to unhealthy, abusive, and exploitative relationships again and again. Because the only thing worse than a bad signal coming in through your aux cord is no signal at all. That's terrifying. That's existential. That's the kind of loneliness and despair that people don't even like to contemplate, and that's exactly where I was.

3

——

TYRONE

My second year with the Los Angeles Rams, John Robinson and the coaching staff who'd drafted me were fired. Suddenly, I had to prove myself to our new coach, Chuck Knox, and his team of assistants. New coaches always come in looking to make tons of changes. Since I was at the bottom of the roster to begin with, I had every reason to be worried. Then, just when I couldn't afford to run into any problems, one of the coaches started harassing me.

His name was Dick Selcer, a little white dude. For whatever reason the guy didn't like me and decided to make me his punching bag. He berated me, dogged me out, called me an idiot on the field, the whole bit. Anytime I so much as thought about standing up for myself, he'd get right in my face and say, "Hey! You come at me, you're going to end up with nothing but an apple and a bus ticket. That's it. The only reason you're here is because somebody up there likes you. But I don't give a damn about you."

One day we were in the meeting room, looking over footage from the practice we'd just completed. I'd had an interception on the field, and it was a fantastic play. Selcer fast-forwarded right past it. The other players noticed. Kevin Greene, the star linebacker at the time, said, "Hey, hey, hey, Terry got an interception. We gotta watch Terry's interception!"

"Ah, it doesn't matter," Selcer said. "He ain't gonna be here anyway."

This guy fucked with my mind in ways that were just bizarre. One day he waved me over and, thinking he was going to tell me something real important, I went to see what he wanted. He pulled out an envelope and showed me a picture of his ass, literally his butt spread wide open. Apparently he'd come from getting a colonoscopy, and he'd decided to use it to mess with me.

"You ever see a pucker like that?" he said. "Huh?!"

"What?!"

"Yeah, man, you ever see an ass like that? Boy, it's beautiful!"

I didn't know what to say. He walked off laughing.

But there was one thing the guy did that made me crazier than anything. One day I heard him calling out on the field, "Hey! Hey, Tyrone!"

I didn't stop, because my name isn't Tyrone, but I saw he kept waving in my direction trying to get my attention. I turned and said, "Hey, man, my name's Terry."

"Nah," he said. "I like Tyrone. From now on I'm gonna call you Tyrone."

And he did. All through training camp, this little white guy kept calling me Tyrone. "Get out there, Tyrone!" "Make it quick, Tyrone!"

There are few things more dehumanizing than not calling someone by their given or chosen name, insisting that they identify as you want to call them. I was a grown-ass man in the NFL, and this guy might as well have been calling me "boy."

The level of degradation was just beyond. It made me seethe with anger. It made me feel so small, but every time he did it, I sucked it up and took it. What I should have done was walk out. I wasn't willing to do that because I was too scared of losing my place on the team. Plus, I was such a pleaser that I still wanted him to like me. Even though anyone could have told me there was nothing I could do to make things right with this guy, I actually told myself, "This is like that movie, *An Officer and a Gentleman*. This is some fucked-up drill sergeant thing where he's trying to break me down to make me into a better player, but when I prove myself and make the team, he's going to come around." So I let it go. Then he cut me anyway.

I was furious. For him to play those games with my head and then kick me out into the street? I called my agent and was like, "What this guy did to me was foul. There has got to be something I can do. Can I sue him?"

My agent just blew me off. "What are you talking about?" he said. "The guy's a coach. Coaches do this all the time."

Now, not only had I lost my place on the team, I'd lost all my self-respect, my entire sense of self-worth. I felt lower than low, helpless and powerless. I could barely talk to Rebecca or even look her in the eye, because I didn't feel like a man anymore. My porn habit was on overdrive. I was going to seedy theaters and video stores, anything to numb the pain I was in. It was as if even the sun didn't shine correctly anymore, and that terrified me.

It started to eat at me that I'd never stood up for myself. All my bottled-up rage started to boil over. It was the closest I've ever come to killing someone. I knew when the team got out of practice at Rams Park, and I mapped out what time I'd need to be there waiting for him. I thought about shooting him but then decided I wanted him to feel it. "I'm gonna chop this dude's head off," I thought. I even knew the knife I was going to do it with—and that scared the shit out of me. It was the same feeling I had the night I beat up my father. Seeing the kind of violence I was capable of terrified me.

As angry as I was with the coach, I was even more pissed off at myself. Because I'd let that guy inside my head. I'd worked my whole life to get to the NFL, only to hand my aux cord to this guy and give him complete control over what I thought and how I felt and how I behaved.

The only thing that saved me in those years was being married to Rebecca. Like that of Mr. Eichelberg and Coach Lee, the input and feedback I got from her was always positive. She looked past all my faults and loved me and believed in me. I should have taken the signal I was receiving from her and turned it up to eleven. I should have let her voice drown out all the others. I didn't, for two reasons. The first was that I was a grade A male chauvinist. I foolishly believed that I was the man and my opinions mattered more than hers— never mind the fact that I didn't really have my own opinions. Whatever other people thought of me was what I thought of myself.

The second reason I didn't listen to her was because the approval I craved was from the same people I'd always craved it from: my parents. I was that little boy, drawing with pencils and crayons and holding up pictures for my mother's approval. Everything I did was to get that reward. It was never simply about the joy of creating or the satisfaction of a job well-done. It was always "Do other people like me? Do the grown-ups approve of me?" In the NFL, the grown-ups were my coaches. By the time I got to Hollywood, the grown-ups were the directors, the producers, and the agents. Honestly, because I was so low on the totem pole, the role of "authority figure" could be filled by just about anyone, because everyone had more status than I did.

As I moved through my early roles in *Training Day* and *Friday after Next*, I was beginning to understand the problem that every performer knows all too well: chasing the high of a great project, only to struggle with the depression that hits after projects are done. I can remember filming *White Chicks* in Vancouver. I was nailing every take. The crew was cracking up on set, and the Wayans brothers were pumping me up every day, telling me what a great job I was doing. After three months of that, I flew back home and I wasn't home two hours when Rebecca asked me to take out the trash—and she didn't applaud for me when I did it, because taking out the trash is just part of the job.

Because I was so dependent on approval from the people above me, I was always racked with anxiety, always petrified that I wasn't doing well enough. Lacking any kind of control over my feelings and emotions at work exacerbated my obsessive need to control everything at home, because I needed to feel in control of *something*. I'd be irritable, short tempered. Honestly, I was mean to my family because I felt that my life had been better in Vancouver when I was filming than it was at home with them. At one point Rebecca even said, "You're nicer when you've got a job."

"I know," I said. "I know. I've got to get back to doing something. I can't not work."

Waiting for *White Chicks* to come out, I would lie in bed for hours. I couldn't make myself get up and do anything, because all I could think about was the big laughs and the opportunities that were going to come once people saw the movie. And the laughs and the opportunities did come. Step-by-step, performance by performance, my career started to take off. But I went through the same spin cycle with every job: the sugar rush of happiness at landing the gig, then the adrenaline wave of working nonstop for three or four months, followed by a major crash and depression when I got home. I became a workaholic. I was always juggling at least two or three projects at the same time, keeping all the plates spinning so that I'd never have a moment of downtime to be alone in my head with no positive feedback coming in. I'd do anything, any project, any role, that someone wanted me to do.

It's no way to build a successful career, but I survived and even thrived for a long time thanks to the benevolent father figures I met along the way. The Wayans brothers, Reggie Hudlin, Chris Rock, Sylvester Stallone, Andre Braugher. I looked up to them and learned from them, and they were all generous and kind and have influenced me in positive ways. But Hollywood has plenty of Coach Thomases and Coach Selcers as well. The ones who aren't outright abusive are merely self-interested; they don't care what's best for you, only what you can do for them. The last thing you want is to be emotionally beholden to those people, but I was.

It was only after D-Day forced me to go into therapy to deal with my sex addiction that I also began to understand my problems with being a pleaser, how it was a common condition among the adult children of addicts and abusers. Talking to my therapist in Phoenix, I was explaining the difficulties I was having with acting. "With my job," I said, "people ask me to do certain things, and I have to do them."

"Why?" she asked.

"Because it's my job."

"But you don't have to do it."

"Yes, I do. It's my job."

She shrugged. "Get another job."

"But I can't get another job," I said. "This is what I want to do."

"So, you want to do it then?"

"No, I have to do it."

"No, no, no, you don't have to do anything," she said. I thought she was doing a Jedi mind trick on me. But she wasn't. She smiled and said, "Terry, you always have a choice. The reason you feel trapped is because you thoroughly believe you have no choice, but you always have a choice. You are the person who decides what you want, not anybody else."

"But what if I lose my job," I said.

"If you lose your job, then that's probably not the job you wanted anyway. There's always another job or another way to do something. If you feel uncomfortable about something or you don't want to do it, you should be able to tell people that."

"But how? I don't know any actors who do that." Then I thought for a moment. "Maybe all of these actors need to be in therapy, too."

"You're right," she said with a laugh, "and half of them are."

It was a funny moment, and as I laughed, her words sunk in, slowly, like water seeping into the ground: we always have a choice. Even if you have a gun to your head, *you have a choice.* We have agency. Every minute of our lives, we can choose how we feel and how we respond to events and what we want to do. We don't always get to choose our circumstances, but we always get to choose what to do with the circumstances that we have.

Up until then, I had always been such a pleaser that I hadn't ever felt I could say no to people. I was too terrified of their disapproval. That was particularly true when it came to figures of power and authority, but it was also true of fans on the street. This image I'd been projecting to the world—big, tough Terry Crews, the king of his castle—none of it was true. I had been utterly powerless my whole life, never deciding my own fate, always reacting to whatever the last person in my ear had told me. I'd never stood up for myself. I had either lashed out in anger or passively followed direction. But I had never been the person in the driver's seat, calmly and methodically steering the course of my own life.

When I came out of therapy in Phoenix, I felt like I was in a whole new world. Literally the first day I was home I stopped at a gas station, and this dude walked up to me. He said he was a fan, and asked if he could take a picture with me. My first instinct was, of course, to say yes, to make sure this guy liked me. But then I caught myself and thought about what I wanted and decided, "No, I'm really not in the mood for this right now."

I looked up quickly and said, "No." I said it real quiet, too, because it felt so strange to say.

"C'mon."

"No," I said, louder this time. "I'm getting gas."

"Come on, man," he said. "Come on."

"NO," I said, practically shouting, really getting into it now. "NO! I'm just pumping my gas. I don't have to give you a picture. I don't owe you anything."

"Dude, forget you, man," he said. "I never wanted it anyway."

When he walked away, I was still pumping my gas, and as I looked around to see if anyone else had noticed what had happened, I realized I was shaking. Being fair to the guy, I had probably taken my new training a bit too far, but after all those years of being the pleaser and going against my own wishes to make everyone else happy, once I started saying no, it felt so good that I couldn't stop. I felt light, full of possibility. I could let go of my compulsion to try to control everything and everyone around me, because I was finally in control of myself.

It was a whole new world.

4

TERRY

On February 4, 2016, Adam Sandler was throwing a party at a restaurant called Hutchinson on La Cienega Boulevard in Hollywood. I was coming off doing two movies with him, *Blended* and *Sandy Wexler*. I was also talking to his company, Happy Madison, about producing a script I'd written. So our relationship was growing, and that was cool, and he invited Rebecca and me to this get-together. Rebecca and I don't normally go to those things, but I decided at the last minute that it would be good to put in an appearance, so we dropped by. It was a packed house, with everyone on the dance floor, and lots of people from that whole Happy Madison, post–*Saturday Night Live* world. Everything was cool. Everyone was having a good time.

We'd been there only twenty minutes when I noticed out of the corner of my eye that a guy across the room was looking and leering at me. He was stocky, around five feet five inches, bald with a goatee, and it looked to me like he was on something, like he was tweaking. He was acting like Tyrone Biggums, that Dave Chappelle crack-addict character. His eyes were all over the place, and he kept sticking his tongue out and wagging it around, the way someone would do if they were pretending to be the devil. It was weird, but no weirder than a lot of shit I've seen in Hollywood. I kept glancing over every few minutes to see if the guy was still looking at me, and he was. Finally, one of my friends noticed my glancing over and said, "That's Adam Venit. Sandler's agent."

I knew who Venit was. He was one of the most powerful people in Hollywood, the head of the film department at my agency, William Morris. My agent at the time, Brad Slater, was always talking about him. I'd done movies with lots of his clients. He represented Sandler, Sylvester Stallone, Eddie Murphy, Gal Gadot, a bunch of people. I had always heard of the guy in passing, but I'd never met him. If I had run into him on the street, I wouldn't have recognized him at all.

Venit started coming over to me with his hand out, and I stuck mine out, too, doing that thing where you're extra friendly with someone to try to keep them at an arm's length.

"Hey, Adam!" I said. "How you doing?"

Then, without warning—no "Hello," no nothing—he reached his hand under mine and grabbed my nuts. I yelled, "HEY!" and pushed him off me into this crowd of people. He sort of wobbled back, got his bearings, and then came back at me and grabbed at my crotch again, hard. It was that way people get when they're drunk or high, where they don't even know how rough they're being.

When he tried to grab me the second time, I pushed him off again, yelling, "YO! What are you doing, man?! Get off me!"

Immediately Rebecca heard me and snapped her head around. "Terry? What is going on with this guy? What's he doing?"

"He's grabbing my nuts, Becky!" I said. "That's what he's doing!"

Venit, after I'd pushed him off the second time, looked at me and started cracking up, "HAHAHAHAHAHAHA!" It was this bizarre, maniacal laughter. Meanwhile, Venit's wife was right next to him. She seemed out of it, too.

People were starting to take notice and stare, and with all those eyes on me, I was keenly aware of how I was being judged. If Adam Venit had done what he did to the old Terry Crews, he might have wound up in the hospital. Stomping a random dude into a Pasadena sidewalk just for brushing my pregnant wife's arm too roughly had nearly cost me everything. Now, after one of the most powerful men in Hollywood had groped me in public, I knew I couldn't respond the same way.

The thing is, I didn't *want* to respond the same way. I knew that my rage had done nothing positive for me my entire life. I knew that anger and toughness of that sort was a symptom of my own weakness and powerlessness. And I knew that if I let Venit make me angry, I would be putting him in control of the situation, and I wasn't about to let him be in control of anything. Once I got past the initial shock of it, I stayed perfectly calm. I went over to Sandler. I didn't raise my voice or lose my temper. I said firmly, "Adam, you'd better go get your boy, because he's gonna get his shit cleaned."

Sandler was like, "What? What's going on?"

"Look at your man!" I said.

Sandler looked over at Venit, who was still acting a fool. "What the fuck is wrong with him?" Sandler said. He said it like, "Hmm, this is so strange and completely out of character for him to act this way."

Sandler and Venit had been buddies for years, so I don't know if Sandler was genuinely shocked to see his boy acting this way, or if he'd seen it before and was acting shocked for my benefit. Either way, I was out of there. Even without the violation of being groped, my normal anxiety and hypersensitivity to being around drunk people was being triggered, too. "I can't stomach this anymore," I told Rebecca. "It's time to go." I grabbed her hand and we got out of there.

Once we got in the car and I was safely away from doing anything stupid inside the restaurant, I finally let my anger out. I was furious. I was screaming in the car, *"How the fuck did this guy do this to me?!"* I couldn't think straight. I wanted to rip the steering wheel off. I wanted to drive back through the club like the Terminator. My mind kept spinning, connecting all these dots trying to make sense of what had happened. "Did Sandler know? Is this why they invited me down here, so they could set me up for this guy and clown me? Was this a joke on me?"

Rebecca kept trying to calm me down. "I'm so proud of you, Terry," she said. "You handled that so well. I'm so proud of you. I'm so proud of you." She kept repeating it the whole way home. We stayed up late and talked about what had happened and what we were going to do about it. I knew I had to do something. I couldn't let it go. But at the same time, I had no idea what my position with William Morris would be if I did. The agency had every reason to protect Venit, and Venit not only represented several people I did business with, he oversaw the whole movie division. Any phone call or movie deal that came in for me, Venit could get in the middle of and cause trouble for me if he wanted to.

The next morning I called my manager, Troy Zien, with 3 Arts Entertainment. I started recounting what had happened, and as I did, I suddenly got a sinking feeling. Because Troy had been recommended to me by Brad, my agent at William Morris. Was Brad going to be on my side in all this, or would he stick by his agency and protect Venit? And if Brad was bringing business to Troy, would Troy be loyal to me or loyal to Brad?

Hollywood is a small town. Everybody's working with everybody. Everybody's got a conflict of interest with somebody else, and everybody's looking out for whatever side their bread is getting buttered on. You have to look hard to find people you can trust, and in that moment I realized I couldn't trust anyone.

When I finished telling Troy what had happened, he said, "Well, you gotta tell Brad." And my thought was "Well, *should* I go to Brad? Is that what I should do? Maybe I should go to the police? Why isn't Troy telling me to go to the police?"

Troy still works with me today, and he's a true friend. But in that moment I doubted him. I was scared to confide in the people I paid to be my confidants. For that to happen to a person like me, someone so other directed that I'd always been driven by the need to please or appease the last person I spoke to, was paralyzing. I got off that phone call with Troy knowing that Rebecca was the only person on earth I could trust. Everything else was just me stumbling around in the dark.

I waited a day, and then decided I should to reach out to Brad. Because I wanted it in writing, I sent him a text: "Brad—your boy Adam Venit—I was hanging with Sandler the other night and he was DOPED UP. It was embarrassing. Sandler had to call me to apologize. He actually grabbed my NUTS. I wish I was making this up. Becky was right there. Somebody need an intervention—QUICK. He almost got knocked out. I kept my peace but I ran outta there. This wasn't drunk bro. I know drunk. It was like bath salts or something."

Brad texted back immediately to say he was calling me . . . from a different phone. So he called me from an outside line and I told him the whole story and he said, "I'm going to talk to Venit. Hold on." A couple of hours later, Brad called back with Venit on the line. Venit was like, "Hey, Terry. Look, I was really drunk and I was out of line and I want to apologize. So, I'm sorry." It was one of those vague, non-apology apologies. Honestly, from the tone of his voice, it sounded like an attorney had coached him on how to sort of apologize without ever admitting to doing the actual thing that he did. It wasn't enough for me, so I pressed him.

"But what was that about?" I said. "How could you think you could do something like that, drunk or not? You think 'I'm sorry' is enough for something like that?" I even called bullshit on the "I was drunk" excuse. "That wasn't alcohol," I said. "That was something else."

"I'm just saying I'm sorry," he said, making it clear that was all I was going to get out of him.

"Okay," I said, and then the call was over.

I called Brad back immediately.

"Is that cool?" he said. "Are you cool?"

"No, I'm not cool," I said. "This is not acceptable. You know something else has to happen."

"Yes, I know," he said, "we're going to do something. There are going to be consequences. Don't worry."

"Okay."

So I waited. For a year. A year went by, and William Morris did nothing. Venit was too powerful. He represented the agency's top clients, all of whom were higher in the pecking order than me. It felt like William Morris was waiting me out, like it was going to memory hole the entire thing and make it seem as if Venit had never done anything to me at all.

As I slowly realized that William Morris wasn't going to do anything to Venit, it also started to sink in what it was going to do to me. From that moment, things got weird with Brad. My career had been going so well with *Brooklyn Nine-Nine*, but now he was sending me these terrible offers, presenting them to me as if they were gold.

Brad also represented Dwayne "The Rock" Johnson, and he offered me an itty-bitty part in Johnson's *Baywatch* reboot. I'd have to

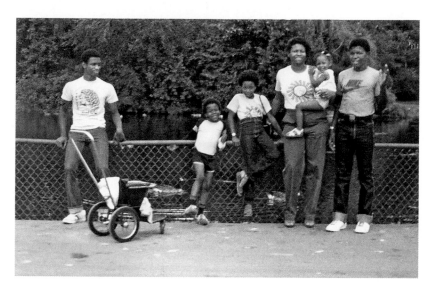

A trip to the Detroit Zoo in seventh grade. (LEFT TO RIGHT): My brother
Marcelle, my cousin A.J., my sister Micki, my mother Trish holding my
cousin Monique, and me; I drew the graphics on the school shirt
my brother is wearing; my design was selected as the official
image on the Holmes Middle School shirt that year.

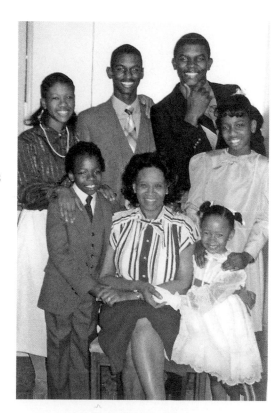

After church on Sunday at
"Mama's" house. (CLOCKWISE
FROM LEFT): Aunt Marketa,
Marcelle, me, Micki,
my cousin Monique,
Grandmother "Mama"
Mary, my cousin A.J.

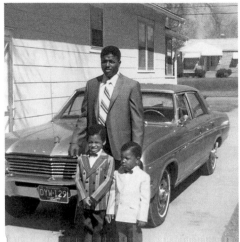

Easter Sunday, on one of the rare occasions my father went to church with us. (LEFT TO RIGHT): Marcelle, Big Terry, and me.

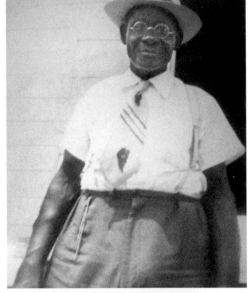

The man, the myth, the legend: Claude Smart.

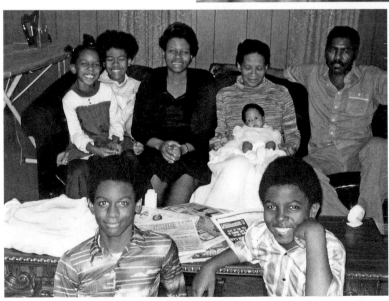

Carol Burnett time at Mama's house. (CLOCKWISE FROM LEFT): Micki, Aunt Marketa, Trish, Mama holding cousin Monique, my stepgrandfather William, me, and Marcelle.

Marcelle holding me
in his lap.

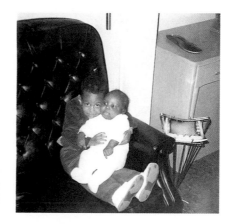

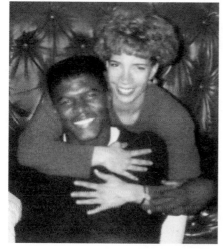

Rebecca and me soon
after we were engaged;
I was nineteen and she
was twenty-one.

Me at six years old,
taking my brand-
new baby sister
Micki to church with
Marcelle and Trish.

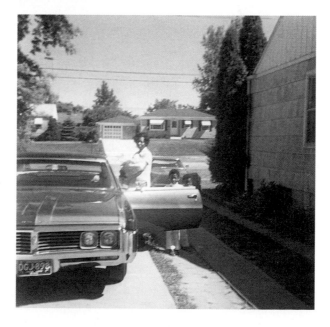

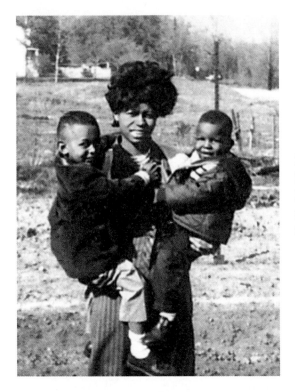

Marcelle, Trish, and me at Mama Z's farm, where we lived during the months my mother moved out from Big Terry.

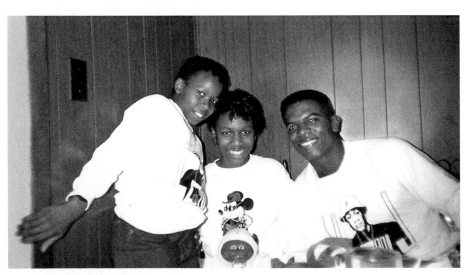

Showing off my T-shirt designs with my cousin A.J. and my sister Micki; a local screen-printing shop called T-Shirts R Us paid me about $25 for each design, and people were wearing my artwork all over Flint without knowing it was mine.

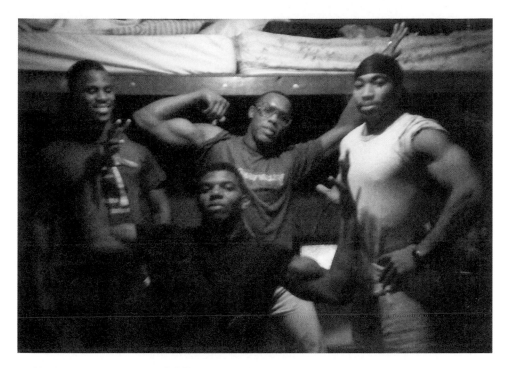

With my suite mates and fellow football players at Western Michigan University.
(LEFT TO RIGHT): Rocky, Arthell, and D.C. I was fresh out of Maranatha Ministries,
and I barely knew them; this was one of the few times we ever hung out.

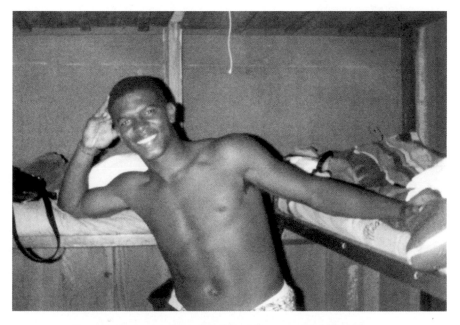

Seventeen years old and having the summer of my life at
Interlochen Arts Camp. Never afraid to go shirtless.

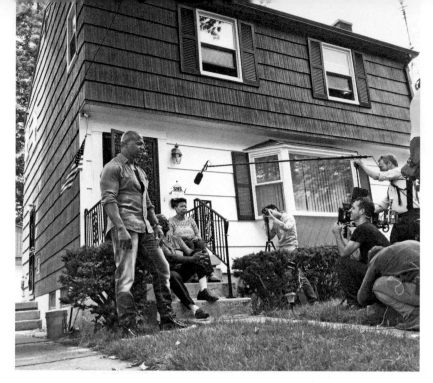

Visiting my mother and father in the house where I spent
most of my childhood; this was the last time I would see
my mother alive, as she died five months later.

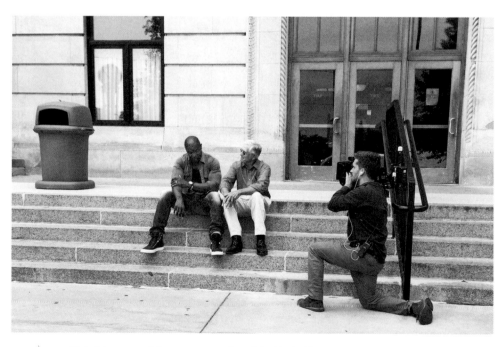

Catching up with my art teacher Mr. Eichelberg on that same trip,
grateful that I got the chance to thank him for believing in me.

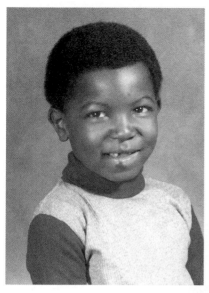

The picture I keep on my desk to remind me I'm still a kid at heart.

In metallic makeup and paint all over for a "robot" performance at a birthday party. I've been performing my whole life.

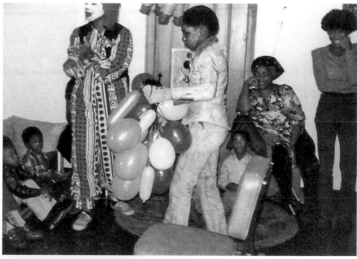

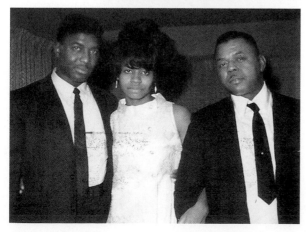

Big Terry and Trish, who was pregnant with me at the time, standing with my maternal grandfather, General Lee Simpson, on the right.

Senior picture fresh, Flint
Academy Eagles, class of 1986.

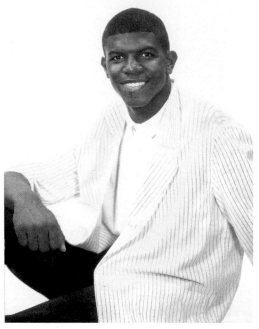

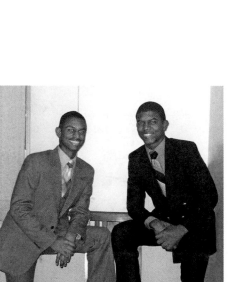

With Marcelle after church; at
fifteen years old, I hadn't grown
into my hands and feet yet.

Goofing around with
Trish and my cousin A.J.,
always trying to make my
mother smile.

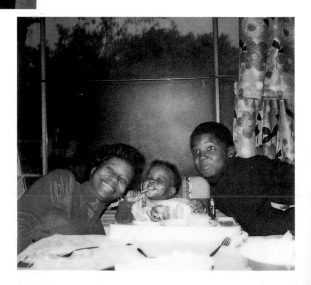

spend two months in Savannah, Georgia, to film it, and the offer was for $75,000. Seventy-five grand was what I'd made on *The 6th Day*, the first movie I ever did back in 1999 when I was a nobody. This was 2017, after I'd accumulated nearly twenty years of experience and notoriety. When I heard the offer, I said, "Huh? Brad, what are you doing, man?"

"It's a great opportunity," he said. "You know, you take less money for the great opportunity."

"But it's not a good opportunity," I said.

He kept spinning all this bullshit that he clearly didn't believe. At that point, I said, "Oh, okay. I see what's going on here."

I fired Brad that day. Then I called Troy and asked him what I should do next. He said I should give Brad another chance, which made me remember that I still couldn't trust Troy, or anybody. However, it was true that I needed to build some new bridges before I burned the old ones. I called Brad and told him I'd give him another chance and stay with him. Meanwhile, I was back to square one trying to figure out what I should do.

Then, on the morning of October 5, 2017, I was sitting on the set of *Brooklyn Nine-Nine*, reading the morning news, and I saw the very first article published about Harvey Weinstein's reign of sexual abuse and harassment in *The New York Times*. In the days that followed, it was like the floodgates opened. Hundreds of women started coming forward about the abuse and harassment they'd suffered not just from Weinstein but from this murderers' row of powerful men across Hollywood and entertainment and nearly every other industry.

Most of the stories I read were newly sympathetic to the women's experiences and perspectives, which had not always been the case. But if you went on Facebook and Twitter, these women were getting dragged by everyone. People were calling them sluts and bitches and worse. People were saying they deserved what they got, that they knew what they were getting into, that women were only saying this stuff now to get money and attention. It was horrible.

Scrolling through all that abuse these women were facing online brought me right back to that night with Venit. The anger and the violation, it all came flooding back. Everybody on set was talking about the articles, and some of the guys were dumbfounded by the extent of the depravity that had been going on, and that's when I told them. "This happened to me," I said. I didn't tell them Venit's name, but I relayed the whole story.

It felt good to get it out. Just like when I came clean to Rebecca about the massage parlor and went public about my pornography addiction, telling the truth felt cathartic. The more I overcame my own shame, the more I talked about those things, the less power they had over me.

The next day, the Weinstein revelations continued to spill out. Everyone was reading them, and I couldn't focus on set. I couldn't concentrate, couldn't get my scenes done. I kept thinking about Venit, about how part of me had wanted to knock him out, even though I knew it would have been a terrible way to respond. Then, on a break between scenes, I looked down at my phone, saw all the Tweets scrolling by, and realized, "Wait a minute. Maybe this is a way to strike back, nonviolently. Maybe this is a way to purge these feelings of anger and shame that I'm carrying around. More important, maybe this is a way for me to support these women." So without telling my agent, my manager, my publicist, or even my wife, I sat down and tweeted out, "This whole thing with Harvey Weinstein is giving me PTSD. Why? Because this kind of thing happened to ME." Then, over a thread of sixteen tweets, I kept going, laying out what had happened, how a high-level Hollywood executive had groped me, how I'd reported it to my agent only to see the issue get buried, the whole story. I concluded by saying, "Hopefully, me coming forward will deter a predator and encourage someone who feels hopeless." I closed my phone and immediately felt relief. I had done something. I had taken the action I needed to take.

I didn't name Venit at first, on purpose. Because I wanted the story to be about what had happened to me, and not about his denial. At the same time, it was my way of putting William Morris on notice: "Y'all motherfuckers know what you did, and now you know I'm not going anywhere."

The whole world changed in that moment. The tweets went viral, and within an hour my phone was blowing up. It was my publicist, my manager, everyone. The first call I picked up was Brad.

"Uh . . . everything okay?" he said.

"No, it's not okay," I said, "and you know exactly who and what I'm talking about."

"Yeah, well . . . ummm . . . so we just want to know if you're okay."

"No, Brad. *I'm not okay.* You guys said you were going to do something, and you never did. It's been a year and no one has ever spoken to me about any kind of repercussions regarding Adam Venit. What are you going to do?"

"I'm going to talk to Ari," he said, meaning his boss, Ari Emanuel, the head of William Morris Endeavor. Ari was out of the country at the moment, but we all agreed to sit down at the Four Seasons Beverly Hills a week or so later and talk things through.

Ari Emanuel's official title is CEO. His actual job description is that he's essentially a pimp. The big lie in Hollywood is that talent agencies work *for* their clients, the actors, directors, and screenwriters. The reality of the business model is that they have a stable of talent that they pimp out to the studios, taking a cut on the back end. Other than a few major movie stars, most of the actors are as interchangeable as the hookers out on the corner. Back in Flint, I'd been around pimps, and the second I sat down with Ari at the Four Seasons, I thought, "Oh, yeah. This guy sounds familiar."

We both sat there and did the requisite small talk to start off. He asked me about working out and intermittent fasting. Then he started talking about alcoholism and drug addiction, how he knew I'd been open about the alcohol abuse in my family and how he'd had family members struggle with that, too. It was all a bunch of manipulative bullshit, trying to forge some kind of fake connection between us to get me on his side, which is what pimps do. "Hey, you know we value you, girl." It was the same thing.

Honestly, it was like meeting with the devil. He struck me as one of the slickest, most arrogant, most manipulative people I'd ever met. He's one of those guys who has that silver tongue, who just knows how to deflect and tell stories and take the conversation exactly where he wants it to go. But I wasn't going to let him. I just looked at him, listened for as long as I felt like it, and then I cut him off.

"I hear you, Ari," I said. "I've got family members on drugs, too. So we've both got family members on drugs. But how are we going to deal with the predator that you have roaming your hallways?"

He talked around in circles for a few minutes, and then I stepped in to cut him off again, saying, "William Morris needs to do something. You guys work for me."

Ari chuckled at that—the same way a pimp would if one of his girls talked back to him. "Lemme tell you what's going to happen," he said. "We're going to demote him and take his title and he's going to be suspended for three months."

"Ari," I said. "You guys have made millions off me, and you're sitting here trying to negotiate why this dude who put his hands on me should stay? It don't work that way at the grocery store, man. If I'm in line and the checkout guy decides to grab my ass, that guy's gone."

"So what do you want?" Ari said.

"I want him gone."

"That's not going to happen."

"Well, then you got a problem."

"Terry, listen," he said. "Venit's a partner, and that's a very difficult situation."

"I don't care," I said. "Being a partner, he should have known better than to put his hands on the clients. It would be different if it had been working the mailroom, but the fact that he's a partner means he's the first one who's supposed to know that."

Ari wouldn't budge, so I took a different tack. Back in 2006, when Mel Gibson had been arrested after going on a sexist, antisemitic tirade, Ari had written an op-ed for the *Huffington Post* about how Hollywood should get rid of Mel Gibson. So I brought that up. "Look here, man," I said. "You wrote this whole thing about Mel Gibson when he went on his antisemitic tirade, about how Hollywood shouldn't put up with it. Now, what Mel Gibson said was reprehensible, but you can't go to jail for it. It's not a crime. Sexual assault is a crime. You go to jail for what Adam did. So you're telling me Mel Gibson deserved to be banished from Hollywood, but what your boy did was okay? Read your own shit, Ari. What you wanted to do to Mel Gibson, that's what should happen to your boy."

"Wow," he said. "I guess we are not going to agree on this. I wish you well."

"All right, man. I'll see you when I see you."

William Morris and I parted ways after that, and from that moment on I was in the wilderness. Rebecca and I were treated like pariahs. Everything went dark and weird. Our close friends stood by us, but all those casual industry acquaintances, all those people who say, "Hey, we should work on something together someday," they all disappeared. The phone didn't ring.

If I was abandoned in Hollywood, online I was attacked. Now it was my turn to get dragged by men, particularly black men. "You should have knocked that white boy out," they'd say. "Terry Crews is a simp. Terry Crews is a pussy. Terry Crews got all that muscle and it ain't meant for nothing. How are you going to let an old white man fondle your balls?" That stuff would get tweeted and retweeted and retweeted, all day long. That was the sports community. That was the rap community. That was everyone.

The irony was that I was being dragged for "not being a man," when I'd actually done the most masculine thing I've ever done in my life. True masculinity, positive masculinity, is using your strength to protect people, to help people. Part of the reason I had to stand behind the women in the Me Too movement was because I could still remember all those nights out with my teammates in the NFL, hearing women saying "No! Stop!," and being too scared to speak up. What kind of man was I that I failed to protect those women back then? I couldn't do that again, especially knowing that I'd been through the same thing. The sad truth of sexism in our society is that women can say the same things a thousand times over and no one will listen, but a man can say it once and the whole world will stop and take notice. I had the power to say something that would help the women brave enough to come forward against Weinstein and the others, and I would have felt like a fraud if I'd stayed silent while those women got publicly stoned.

For the old Terry Crews, the pleasing and appeasing Terry Crews who just wanted to be liked, the whole situation would have been a nightmare, which is why the old Terry Crews probably never would have spoken up in the first place. But I wasn't that guy anymore. Throughout the whole Venit episode, it was like I was a different person from the man I'd been my whole life.

As part of my post-D-Day, self-improvement book-reading binge, one of the most important books I picked up was Viktor Frankl's

Man's Search for Meaning, an account of his time in the Nazi death camp of Auschwitz in World War II. Despite spending years in the camp and losing his entire family, including his wife, Frankl emerged from the war whole. Because he discovered in his experience that even in the most oppressive and brutal experience one might imagine, even with one's whole life stripped away, the Nazi guards could never take away his freedom and ability to decide for himself how to respond to the injustice inflicted upon him. "The experiences of camp life show that man does have a choice of action," he writes. "Man can preserve a vestige of spiritual freedom, of independence of mind, even in such terrible conditions of psychic and physical stress. . . . Everything can be taken from a man but one thing: the last of the human freedoms—to choose one's attitude in any given set of circumstances, to choose one's own way."

I have never endured anything close to what Viktor Frankl endured in the Nazi death camps, but I did endure a childhood of emotional and physical abuse. I put up with years of harassment and humiliation in my career. For years, those experiences filled me up with nothing but anger and bitterness, which I then turned around and inflicted upon my wife and children and others. It was only with the Adam Venit episode that I finally understood what Frankl meant. We should always strive to create a world that is just and fair, but injustice and suffering will always be with us. We cannot will them out of existence, and we cannot control when or how they will be inflicted upon us. We can only control how we respond. Power and agency come from within. Dignity and self-worth come from within. What Adam Venit did to me was wrong, but I can't control the fact that he did it. I can only control how I respond to it.

That is what true power is.

So, despite the fact that I had so much pressure on me to shut up and go away, despite the fact that my entire future in Hollywood was at stake, I knew I couldn't let this pass. As simplistic as it might sound, I knew that no matter what anybody said, no matter what signal was coming in through the aux cord, I needed to stick to my guns and do the right thing. That was my North Star. I locked in on that, and from that moment on I didn't waver.

The first thing I did was file criminal and civil charges against Venit and William Morris. I knew from the jump that the criminal charges weren't going anywhere. When I walked out of the police station after filing them, paparazzi from the gossip website TMZ were waiting for me, which meant someone in the police force was tipping off the media. Then I found out that the event chairman of the Los Angeles Police Foundation, and one of its major donors, was Adam Venit. Like many abusers, he'd spent his whole life cultivating the relationships that he'd need to protect himself if he was ever found out. So from that moment on I knew I couldn't trust the police, and I wasn't surprised when they announced that they wouldn't be pursuing criminal charges.

That left my civil case. As the months passed and the wheels of the legal system slowly began to turn, the entire attitude of William Morris was "Okay, what's it going to take to make this go away? How much money does he want?" But I didn't want money. Because I know that money isn't real. Money is only what it symbolizes, and if I took a payout for my silence, what would that money mean?

I don't mean that as a judgment on any other abuse victim who's taken money in the past. Many of those people, particularly women in show business, were forced to make a brutal calculation. Their careers were effectively over at such a young age, destroyed by the men who wanted them silenced. For them, the money was a life raft they couldn't afford to turn down. I couldn't say the same. Even if I never worked in Hollywood again, I had enough money for Rebecca and me to go and make a new life for ourselves. So for me to take a payoff would have been simply backing down and giving up. I knew what my value was: it was in standing up and telling the truth and trying to have an impact on the culture of Hollywood. I made it perfectly clear: I didn't care what it cost me in attorney's fees. I would spend a million dollars to go to trial to win a dollar in return. All I wanted was for Venit to face real consequences.

When William Morris couldn't come up with a magical figure to buy me off, I believe they were hiring private eyes to go around and dig up dirt on me to try to get me to back off. Which is another reason nobody speaks up about these things. We all have secrets, things we've done that we aren't proud of. Which is why people like Elder Jones accrue so much power, by exploiting our feelings of shame. It's also why there's so much power in letting go of shame. If I hadn't come clean to Rebecca about the massage parlor and the pornography, I probably never would have taken on William Morris. Just the slightest hint that they might dig up my secrets would have whipped me right back in line. But Ari Emanuel couldn't put my shit out there because I'd already put my own shit out there. I'd been on Facebook Live. I'd gone on all the talk shows. I didn't have anything to hide. So when I found out William Morris was digging into my business, I said, "Hey, bring it on. I can do this all day."

Everything William Morris did only strengthened my resolve. When Ari talked down to me like a pimp, it only emboldened me. When the agency tried to buy me off, it only pushed me to go further. I was a man on a mission. Then, that January, I was at the Sundance Film Festival when a man approached me. I can't say his name, but he's someone I know through different projects I've done. "Venit did the same thing to me," the guy said. "I can't go public because of my family, but I'd like to join your case privately."

He was the first. In the months that followed, my attorney and I were contacted by four more, all of them sharing stories of sexual assault at the hands of Adam Venit. They all agreed to help with the case. Now I knew I could never back down. I wasn't just on this mission for myself, and I wasn't fighting on behalf of sexual abuse survivors in general. I had five people counting on me to see this through, none of whom would have been powerful enough to stand up to Venit on their own.

That April we finally got to sit down for arbitration. My one sticking point was that Venit be terminated, which was the one thing William Morris refused to do. The agency dug in its heels and was ready to go to war, and then we put the testimony of the other accusers on the table. Now it wasn't just a "he said, he said." It was a pattern of abuse going back years. William Morris couldn't wave the white flag fast enough. It wanted this over and done. Venit was required to resign as part of the settlement. I'd spent nearly half a million in attorney's fees, and I got every penny reimbursed. Most important, William Morris had to agree to put real accountability measures in place. What had happened to me, where I informed my agent of what Venit had done only to see the matter get buried? William Morris can't let that happen again. If it does, it'll face real legal consequences.

A couple of months later, I was contacted by Amanda Nguyen. She's a Nobel Peace Prize nominee and a Harvard graduate. She's also a rape survivor. Amanda asked me to join her on Capitol Hill to speak to a Senate committee on behalf of the Sexual Assault Survivors' Bill of Rights, which she was trying to push into law. Amanda told me she wanted me to testify because she knew that no matter how many women came before the committee, if she had one man, people would pay that much more attention, especially if that man was a celebrity.

I accepted the invitation. The day I went to Congress to testify, it was standing room only. For a kid from Flint, Michigan, to be the subject of a packed Senate hearing was unreal. It was the moment when I realized how far my own experience went beyond me. What had started with "I'm going to show Ari Emanuel that he's not going to get away with this" had become part of a larger crusade on behalf of any and every person who's ever suffered sexual abuse.

The moment from the hearing that went viral online was Senator Dianne Feinstein asking me the same question everyone else on social media had been asking: "Why didn't you just knock the guy out?" The obvious part of the answer is that I knew, as a black man, what would happen to me if I did. I'd have been arrested. But the deeper answer is that rage and anger are never the way. Anytime you're acting out of anger, you are not in control. You're allowing yourself to be provoked. To be filled with anger and rage is to be powerless and weak.

When I die and people take the measure of my public life, everything I've done outside of being a husband and a father, I feel—or at least I hope—that my decision to stand up against sexual abuse will be remembered as the most important thing I ever accomplished. Not simply for what I did but for how and why I did it. The whole time, I was never angry. I was never driven by rage. I was controlled, thoughtful, methodical. It was the polar opposite of the way I reacted to every other abuser I'd had in my life. I'd always bottled everything up. I'd always been consumed by feelings of powerlessness that boiled over into rage—rage that was typically unleashed on anyone other than my abusers. All those other times with Coach Selcer and the church and growing up, I was always reacting to someone else's decisions. Not anymore. I knew what I was doing. I was in complete control. For the first time in my life, I saw myself as powerful. I saw myself as having true agency.

Letting someone else make you angry is giving them too much control over your life. You cannot control what happens to you, but you can always control how you respond. You are never powerless. You always have a choice. Anytime anybody tells you that you don't have a choice, they're already deciding for you. It's one thing to hand a passenger the aux cord to let them control the mood in the car; it's another thing to move over, give them the wheel, and let them drive. That's what I'd been doing my whole life. Now, through the painful Adam Venit affair, I had finally come 180 degrees from how I'd let myself and others treat me. It was so amazing to see myself for who I really was.

V

IDENTITY

1

INTERLOCHEN

My art teacher in high school was a guy named Mr. Eichelberg. White guy. Very white. When he wasn't teaching
he was a corn farmer out in rural Michigan; he used to
bring us fresh corn to class.

Mr. Eichelberg was the guy who always used to encourage me to
be an artist. "Terry," he'd say, "you're the best artist I've ever taught.
The work you're doing right now, I can't even do. You have a talent
that I've never seen."

For a long time I didn't believe him. Sometimes I even thought he
was putting me on. I felt that in part because I was so hard on myself. I wanted my work to be perfect. I'd spend hours on a painting,
going late into the night, obsessing over every detail. When I finally
went to bed, I'd think, "This is awesome." Then, as soon as I woke up
in the morning, I'd think, "This is horrible." I could only see what
was wrong with it.

Another reason I didn't believe him was that my mother had done so much to cripple my self-confidence, always calling me stupid and making me feel worthless. But the biggest reason I didn't believe Mr. Eichelberg was because I was black. It wasn't Mr. Eichelberg who made me feel that way; he was nothing but supportive. But I would look out at the lily-white world of fine art, and I never saw the work of people like me hanging on the walls at MoMA or the Guggenheim. I felt like my being black meant there was something about being an artist that I didn't understand and would never understand. It just wasn't where I belonged.

Then, my senior year, Mr. Eichelberg did two things that changed my life. First, without even telling me, when he heard I was going to Western Michigan, he took pictures of my work and submitted them with an application for me to get the art scholarship that paid part of my tuition and allowed me to go. Then, after he did that, he applied for and got me a full-tuition grant from the Chrysler Corporation to attend a six-week summer program at the Interlochen Arts Academy in northern Michigan.

I flipped when he told me. Interlochen was, and still is, one of the most prestigious art schools in the world. As it turned out, Interlochen would also be my first experience with entering an all-white world, which was . . . wow. My buddy Ron Croudy had been awarded a slot, too, and he and I arrived to find that, out of maybe 2,500 kids, we were two of only a handful of black students there.

That cultural imbalance led to some awkward moments, of course, but fewer than you'd think. We were all there because we had something in common that transcended the way we looked. Also, no amount of tension or awkwardness could dampen the incredible experience of being there. I got to be outside and play and draw and paint and have fun. We had a big old VHS camera that we used to make videos and short movies. We were nowhere near the city lights, and at night the stars would come out. We would lie on our backs and look up, and it felt like we were falling in the sky. After all the darkness of growing up in Flint, it was extraordinary. I can't even describe it; it was bliss. There was no abuse, no alcoholism, no shootings; the only big drama was that two kids got caught making out in a tuba locker.

Interlochen also gave me an experience that changed my life. In my drawing class, we had been doing still lifes in charcoal. Each student had to submit two pieces to be judged in a competition, and they were submitted anonymously so the judging would be objective. Since there were about twenty kids in the class, that meant about forty works in the competition—various paintings of pottery and bowls of fruit and that sort of thing.

The judge was a professor from the Art Institute of Cincinnati. We all stood in the back, nervous, as he walked down the gallery of work. He did one pass and then went right back to the first of my two paintings. "This," he said, "is the best one in the class." Then he walked all the way across the room to the other work I'd submitted. "And this," he said, "is the second best."

I was like, "Holy shit . . . I'm the best one here."

And it wasn't just American kids in the class. There were students from Germany and Italy and all over the world, the best of the best of the best, and when my name was revealed as the artist behind the two winning pieces, they all burst into applause. *For me.* After eighteen years of being told, both explicitly and implicitly, that being black made me somehow inferior, that was the first moment in my life where I felt that I was as good as everybody else, no matter what color my skin was or how I spoke or what neighborhood I came from. It was euphoric, and I've been chasing that high ever since.

2

TWO MICHIGANS

The first time I got called a nigger was in fourth grade. We'd just moved to Civic Park. The neighborhood was flipping, but there were enough white kids around that they felt like it was still their turf. One day on the bus, a white kid who was older than me stood up and turned around and, literally out of nowhere, called me a nigger. All of the kids around us were like, "Oooooooh," watching and waiting to see what I would do. Since it was mostly white kids on the bus, I didn't do anything. I ignored it.

When we got off the bus, he followed me, and he kept saying it. "I'm gonna kick your ass, nigger!" Then his brother came up behind him, getting in on it. I kept walking and saying, "Man, forget you." Then I heard "Hey!" real loud. I turned around and *POW!* The dude coldcocked me dead in the face. I saw lights and went down, and he jumped on me and kept pounding on me, yelling, "Fuckin' nigger! Fuckin' nigger!"

The thing is, being a kid, I was more confused than insulted. The experience didn't make sense because I couldn't put it together, meaning the slur and me. I knew what "nigger" meant, and I knew who Terry Crews was, and I knew Terry Crews wasn't a nigger. So it didn't compute, and because it didn't compute, I didn't know to be insulted. I had plenty of other insecurities that kid might have teased me for, but being a black kid on a white bus wasn't one of them.

An insult hurts only if there's a ring of truth to it; it only hurts if you believe it. My mother calling my dad a broke-ass drunk cut him to the bone, because it was true. But if you called Bill Gates broke, you wouldn't be insulting the man, because he knows he isn't broke. He'd laugh at you and shrug it off. That's how I felt walking away from the bus that day. I didn't like that I'd gotten my ass kicked, but that kid didn't hurt my feelings by using that word. Nobody's ever hurt me by using that word, because I've always known that that word has nothing to do with who I am.

I don't know where that confidence came from, because it didn't come from my mom or my dad, that's for sure. Just like my parents taught me nothing about sex or money, they taught me nothing about race, nothing about what it meant to be a black man in America. Our family's past, growing up in Jim Crow Georgia, it wasn't talked about. It was too painful. The little I did learn I picked up along the way, like the fact that my father's grandfather, Claude Smart, worked on one of the construction crews that built Fort Benning. As the story goes, one day his bosses made him go out and work in the middle of a thunderstorm, and he got struck by lightning. "Shocked out of his shoes," people used to say, conjuring an image of an empty pair of rubber boots smoking on the ground. But that isn't even the crazy part of the story. The crazy part is that once his bosses realized he wasn't dead, they made him get back to work.

"You okay?"

"Yeah, I made it."

"Okay, get back out there."

Such was life for a black man in Georgia at the time—get hit by lightning, and then get your ass back out there.

As for how our families got to Michigan as part of the Great Migration out of the South and slavery and all the rest of it, I learned that on my own or in school, where we got the usual storybook lessons about Harriet Tubman and Rosa Parks and Martin Luther King Jr., and not much else.

If my parents were loath to bring up the past, they weren't too keen on discussing the present, either. My mom lived in the bubble of the church, rarely crossed the color line, and rarely brought up the subject of white people at all. As for my father, he was always a loner and an outcast, always out of step with the zeitgeist. He didn't march in the sixties. His ticket out of Georgia had been the military, so he was a big military guy. You keep your head down and work. That was his whole thing.

By the time I was coming up, it was the peak of the Hollywood Blaxploitation era. All these guys were coming back from Vietnam with big Afros and bell bottoms talking all this jive about black power. My dad *hated* that. And of course when hip-hop came around, my dad was that old guy sitting in his chair, going, "These niggas need to pull their pants up."

At the General Motors shop, my dad was even more out of step. The truth about Michigan is that there are two Michigans. There's black Michigan and there's white Michigan. There's Detroit inside 8 Mile, and there's Detroit outside 8 Mile. There's Flint and there's Ann Arbor. At GM, both Michigans had to work together, but the factory was run like a prison. It had gangs. There was the black gang and the white gang, and my father wasn't a part of either.

As one of, if not the only, black foremen in the shop, he wasn't out on the floor with all the black laborers; in fact, he was often at odds with them over different workplace issues. But instead of that difference being a bridge across the color line, it became another point of division. The black laborers looked at him as a sellout, and he looked at them like the reason they weren't successful was because they were lazy. "These niggas just don't wanna work," he'd say. But even as he was ostracized from the black gang, he was never actually welcome in the white gang. The other managers who should have been his peers and colleagues never invited him to happy hour, never invited us to their Fourth of July barbecues.

My father never moved up out of middle management—and that, really, was the only lesson he ever taught me about race. Anytime I'd talk about my big dreams of going to Hollywood or making movies, he'd say, "The white man is only going to let you get so far." He'd say it like he was helping me, keeping it real with me, teaching me not to get my hopes up so I wouldn't be disappointed. His only advice was to go into the military, because that was the one place a black man would be protected. And that was everything I learned at home on race. My mom taught me to pray for a better life in the next world, and my dad taught me to accept the limitations of this one. It's no surprise I didn't think I was good enough to go to a place like Interlochen.

The messages I absorbed about race out in the world weren't too different from what I was learning at home. I loved *Star Wars* and sci-fi, but until Lando Calrissian showed up, it generally seemed as if black people didn't even exist in the future. I'd flip my TV to *The Brady Bunch* and the family would be in Hawaii, because every show had to have a Hawaii episode back then. Little Cindy Brady would be getting this big glass of milk for breakfast, and I'd be like, "Woooo, they gave that white girl all that milk?! She'd better not waste a drop of that." All the white people on television were living good, and we weren't living good—and the only message to take away from that was that we had to be doing something wrong.

In the beginning, the world outside my door wasn't too bad. Flint was still booming. The white people hadn't left for the suburbs yet. I'd go down the street and play with Ricky and Danny. My elementary school was mixed and everybody got along. My first-grade teacher was a blond white lady named Mrs. Sullivan, and she was the nicest woman. I don't remember her or anyone else ever treating me any different because I was black.

Then came seventh grade. That's when everything changed. The gas crisis hit and the factories started to close and, other than old Mrs. McCauley next door, white people couldn't get out of there fast enough. As the city started to crater, the newspapers salivated over every detail. If it bled, it led, and if a black man was responsible for it, all the better. Anytime a black man did anything, the headlines would literally read A BLACK MAN KILLED THREE PEOPLE TODAY or BLACK MAN HAS CRACK DEN or FOUR DEAD IN CRACK DEN, WITH SEVERAL BLACK PEOPLE. If it was a white man, he was just a man, but if it was a black man, his race was always called out. Now, imagine reading that as a thirteen-year-old black boy who was in the process of becoming one of those black men.

Seventh grade was the year I went from being treated like a black boy to being treated like a black man, and the difference was stark. I noticed it the minute it happened. My mother loved going to the big department stores at the mall. As a kid, I hated it because she would spend all her time trying stuff on but then never buy anything because we didn't have any money. As an adolescent, I hated it because I had white salespeople on me all the time. "What do you want? What are you looking for? What do you need? Can I help you?" Even after they backed off, I could feel their eyes following me around the store, like I was about to steal something.

Even well-meaning white people used to say things to me like

"You're a good kid, Terry. Don't become a criminal." I would stare at them, like, "Criminal? What are you talking about? I'm twelve."

I spent my whole childhood always navigating between the Two Michigans. For football and basketball, we used to take a bus to play at schools in the suburbs, and we'd always stop at McDonald's after the games. We would get off the bus and go in, and the minute we walked through the door, all the white people would stop eating and look at us. We knew enough not to eat inside. We'd get our food and get back on the bus and eat there. It was too awkward to sit inside with everyone staring at us.

Back in the black neighborhoods of Flint, there was a different problem. Juice and the other Top Dawgs were always hanging around on the street right outside. I didn't dare walk with my white friends to the bus for the looks and the barrage of insults I'd get hurled at me. "What's up, white boy?" and "Oh man, you talkin' all white. Look at you tryin' to sound all proper." I never understood it. I was always like, "How do you 'talk white'? I'm just talking."

I hated the walk home from school. I had to learn to avoid eye contact, because young dudes would be staring me down, and if I looked at them wrong, they might kill me. Young black men in Flint were getting murdered every day. Whenever I was outside of school, I had to adopt this pose. I'd be putting on exaggerated black slang and acting "more black" just to go along, otherwise I'd get ostracized, or worse, for hanging with white kids and being "too white."

The whole thing was ridiculous to me, because unlike most of my peers, I'd actually left Flint. I knew there was no one way to be "authentically black." For one week every summer my dad used to take us down to visit our relatives in Edison, Georgia. It was always a huge culture shock for me because it was so rural, staying in my grandmother's tiny house with no TV, no air-conditioning, and nothing to do except "go outside and play" in the blazing hot sun baking into the red clay dirt.

Me and my cousin Colby were the same age. We'd be out in the yard, and we'd always fight because of the cultural divide between us. It was always an "up North, down South" thing. Colby's family was real country. All their music was from four or five years back. We thought they were backward, and they thought we were uppity. A lot of it had to do with culture, but even more, it was about the way we spoke. They always used to say to me and my brother, "You guys talk funny," and we'd be like, "You talk funnier."

So every summer, being a black kid from the streets of Flint made me the wrong kind of black person to my cousins down south. Then, back in Flint, being a black kid from a magnet school made me the wrong kind of black person to the other kids in the street. I experienced that stuff my whole life, and it was dumb to me even then. There is no right way to be black or white or anything else. There are literally thousands of different ways to be in this world, so ultimately all you can be is yourself.

Luckily for me, there were two Terrys to go with the two Michigans. I was a nerd who was into art, but I was also an athlete who was jacked. That was the only thing that saved my life, because sports coded as black. Out in the streets, my varsity jacket made me black enough to get a pass I wouldn't have gotten otherwise. Having some neck on me didn't hurt, either.

Actually being at school was an oasis. Inside Flint Academy, among the students, it wasn't like that at all. There were still two Michigans, for sure, but the borders were broken down, and people moved freely back and forth. We had black kids assimilating with the white kids, but we also had white kids assimilating with the black kids. When Eminem came along as this black-talking white boy in the nineties, people looked at him as an anomaly. But back in the day we had fifty Eminems. I still remember my man Matejik. He was a straight-up white boy, and he had a Jheri curl. He'd be in the men's room literally spraying in curl activator right along with the black guys. We had white girls with Jheri curl, too; their hair would look wet the whole day.

By senior year, my three best friends were three white girls. I had secret crushes on each one of them at one time or another, but since I wasn't allowed to date, it never became a thing, racial or otherwise. They were all one grade lower than me, and we sat at lunch together every day and it was no big deal. It wasn't some post-racial utopia; kids had issues here and there. But by and large we were just organically doing what the whole civil rights movement had fought for us to do: getting to know each other across the color line and learning how to move on from the past.

The only ones who didn't get the memo were the faculty. Unlike Mr. Eichelberg, some of the faculty, both white and black, were too old and too stuck in the past to adapt to the new reality that was in front of them. In middle school, I got Mr. Krabill, an old white guy with horn-rimmed glasses. Mr. Krabill laid out his class seating chart from smartest to dumbest—and I'm not kidding. After every test score, he'd put out a new list of seating assignments and you'd have to go find your new one. Whoever had the best score would get the first seat in the front row. Then it would go down in descending order to the lowest in the back. Of course, because all the black kids were being funneled in from the worst elementary schools, the front rows of the classroom were always all white, while the back rows were always almost all black. You couldn't help but feel less than. Anytime I asked a question, Mr. Krabill used to look at me like I was an idiot, like I was a waste of his time.

On the other hand, there was my senior guidance counselor, a black woman. One day she saw me in the hallway and waved me down. "Terry," she said, "do you have a moment? I've got something very important I need to tell you."

"Okay," I said.

She turned and I followed her back to her office, thinking, "Oh my god. I must have gotten a scholarship to one of the colleges I applied to." Then, when we got to her office, she closed the door, asked me to sit down, and said, "Terry, what I'm about to tell you is important. It's going to affect your life forever."

"Okay."

"And I want you to hear me because it's very important that you listen to me and follow my instructions."

"Oh, man. Okay. What is it?"

"Stay away from white women."

I stared at her. "Excuse me?"

"Terry, listen to me, they will be your downfall. They will stop anything you want from happening in your life. They will be the reason you fail."

"Huh?"

"You have to stay away from white women. They will be the end of you."

"O-kay. Thanks!"

"Do you hear me?"

"Mmm-hmm."

"Do you understand what I'm telling you?"

"Yes, ma'am."

I didn't even argue with her. I wanted to get out of there and have the conversation be over. I thought it was the most ridiculous thing I had ever heard, even at the time. There are those who say that black people can't be racist, but I'm sorry: that woman was racist. She was no different from Juice and his boys out in the street, trying to tell me how to be black.

But out of everything that happened to me as a black kid growing up, the one thing that stands out in my mind nearly forty years later isn't being called "nigger" or getting beat up by white kids on the bus. It's something far more subtle. In high school, I had an assistant coach, a white guy, Mr. Scanlon, who'd gone to the University of Michigan, which has one of the best teams in college football. He knew I wanted to play football at a Division I school and then go on to the NFL, so one day when I was fifteen he offered to take me down to Ann Arbor for a game.

Ann Arbor was like heaven—stately avenues, gorgeous houses, every tree and lawn trimmed and manicured. Mr. Scanlon took me to a big alumni tailgate party. There was all this food, and he was introducing me around, going, "This is my student, Terry." I was shaking hands with everybody. Then we went to the game and I was there with over one hundred thousand people in the stands and Michigan won and the whole place went nuts and I sat there like, "Holy cow! This is *amazing*!"

On the drive home, I was so excited. "You know what, Mr. Scanlon?" I said. "I'm going to Michigan!"

"What?" he said.

"I am *going* to Michigan. This is where I want to play."

"Terry," he said, shaking his head, "you can't do that."

"Huh, what do you mean?"

"Terry, I gotta be honest with you, I don't think you're Michigan material. The competition is huge. You want to go where you could thrive. Maybe go to junior college for a couple of years, and then you can look at something else for year three. But I don't see you going to Michigan."

I stared at him like, "Well, why the fuck did you take me to Michigan then? What the fuck was this? Why would you take me here? Why would you even show me this?"

All of a sudden, the whole day played back in my head, his introducing me to everybody like he was so proud of me. That's when I
realized, "Oh, he was just showing me off." Like he wanted brownie
points for adopting the little ghetto kid for a day. Like I was a rescue
dog from the pound or something, and wasn't he a good guy for helping me out. I was furious. He dropped me off at my house, and I got
out the car and didn't even say goodbye. And that moment flipped a
switch in me. From that day on, my attitude was "Fuck that guy. I'll
show him. I'll show everybody." I fed on that memory for years. It
struck a spark of anger and resentment in me that I'd never had as
a kid, even with everything I went through, and that anger carried
me all the way onto the field at Western Michigan.

3

TRAPPED

When I got to college, the first racism I encountered was in the athletic system. It was on full display. The coaches didn't even hide the fact that they didn't care about my education. I wasn't there to learn. I was the big black kid who was there to play football—for *them*. When my grades started to suffer because I couldn't afford the art supplies I needed to complete some of my assignments, the coaches told me I should go be a business major so I could continue to play, which pissed me off.

It also didn't take long to notice that they played all the white guys in what they called the "thinking man's positions." Meanwhile, the black players were just out there on the field to be enormous pieces of meat. I was stuck playing defensive end. I knew I should have been playing linebacker, but I had a coach flat out tell me I wasn't smart enough to play linebacker, never mind the fact that I would later go on to be a linebacker in the NFL for seven seasons.

One year we had a brilliant quarterback, but he was black. These were the days before white people could fathom the thought of a black quarterback, so the coaches made him the backup. They started a little white freshman from Canada instead. The little white freshman *led the nation* in interceptions, but they stuck with him while the brilliant black quarterback sat riding the bench.

That's the way it was. The coaches treated black players like we were animals, and most of us were angry as a result. A few years after I left, the black players actually got together and staged a sit-down strike where they refused to even go out on the field because of the discrimination they felt. But at the time we didn't feel there was anything we could do. It was the hand we'd been dealt and it was our only ticket to the NFL and we couldn't mess it up. So we took what we were given.

Being black off the football field was a completely different set of challenges. The campus of Western Michigan was extremely segregated, and I actually didn't fit in with most of the black people there. The hub of black social life on campus was the black fraternities, and it all centered on drinking, which I still couldn't handle. The hazing was unreal. It was brutal. I watched guys go through pledge week and come out bleeding, bruised, beat up, starved, made to stay awake for days at a time. It was not good; the whole scene reminded me of the Young Boys back home.

I also didn't like the segregation of the Greek system as a whole. There were black fraternities and white fraternities and nothing in between, nothing like the integrated oasis I'd enjoyed at Flint Academy. I knew I wasn't welcome at the white fraternities, but the vibe at the black fraternities wasn't welcoming, either.

The 1970s had seen the rise of the whole Black Power, Black Is Beautiful movement. It was never talked about in my house because of my parents, but I understood where it came from. Black people had been excluded from public life and popular culture for so long, and then a movement came along to say, "Hey, we're here. We belong in the American story, too. We matter." For people who'd been made to feel so unworthy for so long, Black Power was a long-overdue assertion of self-worth. But any social movement, no matter how well intentioned, can lose its way. Any philosophy, no matter how just, can be twisted by unscrupulous people into something else. Jesus preached nothing but love and humility and grace. But Elder Jones took that gospel and used it to build a sexually repressive and emotionally debilitating cult that robbed my mother of her life.

By the time I got to college, Black Power had long since curdled into something else. All identity is performative to some degree, but some people were taking it to the level of parody. Things had become very ethnocentric. Lots of leather Africa medallions, Public Enemy swag, kente cloth everything. Kids had red, black, and green flags up in their dorm rooms. It was all very "Look at me and how black I am."

Because black Americans had been robbed of our heritage by slavery, there was also a strange thing of people going around and making shit up to fill in the gaps of what we didn't know, all this Afrocentric jive about black people being descended from Egyptian kings and queens. Usually it was some older dude who'd never graduated but was still hanging around campus. He'd go around preaching that stuff. "My brother, you are a king. You are descended from kings."

Anytime any black guy starts a sentence with "my brother," you can be sure what's coming next is going to be nonsense.

Most college students go through different phases, trying on extreme personas, wearing their identity on their sleeves, so that element of it wasn't a big deal, and the ridiculous parts of it were easy to dismiss, but the dangerous undercurrent was that a lot of it was pro-black to the point of being anti-white. Everything was us versus them, and you're either with us or against us. You couldn't admit to watching *Saturday Night Live*, only *In Living Color*. Hip-hop, which had started out a very multicultural art form in the streets of the Bronx, was now almost exclusively the voice of angry black youth. Everything was about race, and everything *had* to be about race.

One thing you learn as you get older is that most of life is not about race. There's nothing "black" or "white" about replacing your car battery or teaching your kids how to tie their shoes, and that's what most of life is, day to day. But when you hang your whole identity on race, you have to attach the word "black" to everything, because anything that isn't black, by definition, is white, and anything that's white is bad and doesn't include us. So there couldn't just be "economics" or "math." It had to be "black" economics and "black" math. Every year, students and professors were protesting on campus, demanding that all this be taught in black studies.

I took a few of those courses, and it wasn't at all what I expected. What I thought I was signing up for were classes that corrected the whitewashed version of American history that left black people out. I wanted to know where my family came from, the real history of slavery and Jim Crow. Certainly, by the late 1980s, there were many black academics engaging in that kind of rigorous scholarship at colleges across the country, but that's not what I got in the classes I took. What I got was a bunch of dubious claims about "whiteness" and "blackness." Some of the professors took it to the point where they were talking about black people and white people as if we were two different species. It was "white people spend money like *this*," and "black people spend money like *this*," and the subtext running through all of it was that whatever the black people were doing was better. "Eurocentric" culture was cold and patriarchal and exploitative. "Afrocentric" culture was warm and tribal and loving. It was like somebody had taken a bunch of stereotypes like "white men can't jump" and "black people are better at dancing" and tried to turn them into a philosophy.

I even had people I trusted and loved try to give me the ridiculous "melanated" conversation. How the melanin of black people makes them more compassionate and loving, and a white person's lack of it makes them calculating and cruel. "White devils" they were called. It was nothing more than the inverse of the same scientific racism that was used to justify slavery. James Baldwin had a name for it. He used to call it "mystical black bullshit," and I couldn't agree more. I used to sit in those classes thinking, "This is ridiculous." Because it wasn't true to my experience. Yeah, I'd had white kids beat me up and call me a nigger, but I'd also had white teachers like Mr. Eichelberg nurture me and lift me up. I'd had black people like Mama Z who were warm and loving, but I'd also had black people like Juice and the Top Dawgs who were the complete opposite of that. Ultimately, any philosophy that painted "whiteness" and "blackness" into these cartoonish categories, I just couldn't go along with.

On the one hand, with hindsight, I understand why all of this was happening and why so many of my fellow black students were swept up by it. The oppression of black people in America had been so extreme for so long, the pendulum was bound to swing to similar extremes when it went the other way. On the other hand, if you replace one falsehood with another falsehood, you haven't exactly achieved truth. You cannot swap the lies of white supremacy with lies about melanin and Egyptian kings and claim that you've made progress.

I wasn't the only black student who felt that way, of course. But among the black minority it was by far the dominant culture on campus at the time. You didn't dare raise your hand in a black studies class to say, "Well, actually I went to an integrated school and I got along fine and most of the teachers were great." Hell, no. Try that and it'd be "You're an Uncle Tom" and "He's a sellout," and you'd never hear the end of it.

Which didn't leave me a whole lot of options, socially. If you weren't a part of Greek scene or the black studies crowd, what you had left was mostly white kids. Hanging with white kids had never been a problem for me in high school, but the white kids I knew at Flint Academy had been forced to develop at least some proficiency with race to get along in an integrated crowd. Most of the white kids at Western Michigan were painfully naive. They'd come from lily-white suburbs or small towns up North where black folks only lived across the railroad tracks, if there were even any black folks at all.

That was the type of white kid that I encountered at Maranatha. Maranatha was a small group, about twenty-five students. Maybe three of us were black. The pastors were always looking to expand that. They wanted to get more black people in, and by black people they meant "the right kind of black people," role model types like student leaders and student athletes. When they got me to join, they made a big deal of the fact that A. C. Green from the LA Lakers was in the church. That really hooked me, because it made this seem like the club I wanted to belong to. Once I joined, I quickly became their go-to for recruiting other black kids. I was an art major, came from a magnet school, didn't drink, played football. They loved to show me off as their "black guy."

It's painfully obvious in hindsight that I was being used, but I'll be honest. In the beginning it felt good to be held up in a positive way because so few people in my life had ever treated me with any kind of appreciation. But pretty quickly the naivete of the white pastors and students started to show. They had no gauge for how to talk to me. If we were having a picnic or a potluck, they'd always over-emphasize whatever they thought was black about it. "Ohhhh, Terry, we're gonna have a *soul food* cookout tonight! There's gonna be *ribs*. Don't you just love *ribs*?! How about some *mac and cheese*?"

When they told me I had to get rid of my hip-hop tapes because Jesus wouldn't listen to that kind of music, they went out and bought me cassettes tapes from all these Christian rappers that the church recommended. They were . . . not good. *"We love Jesus, yeah, yeah, yeah! One! Two! Three! He's the one for me!"* It was so horrible, and all the white people would look at me like, "Isn't this *great*!" I learned to nod and smile, and they'd be happy that I was happy.

I wouldn't say that I enjoyed it; it was a barrier to ever forming real relationships with those people. But I never called them on it, either, because it didn't bother me. Other people's ignorance, about race or anything else, has never bothered me, because ignorance is something people often can't help. It's the same as how being called nigger doesn't land on me, either; that I can brush off. But what pissed me off then and what pisses me off to this day is people putting limitations on who I am and what I can do. Anything that triggers memories of my mother calling me stupid, my father telling me what the white man won't let me do, or my coach telling me I couldn't go to Michigan—that shit drives me up the wall. I cannot abide anyone telling me that my blackness puts limits on where or how high I can go.

Of course, at the same time, I didn't feel like there was anywhere I *could* go. When I looked behind me to Flint, all I saw was a place that was dying. Many of my friends were getting killed in the streets. Most of the others were going to jail. One of my best buddies from elementary school all the way up throughout high school ended up on crack. I remember running into him, and he had these black lips and was rail thin. I was like, "Hey, man!" and he looked at me like he was a zombie.

I knew I could never go back, but when I looked ahead, all I could see was a world that wanted me to know my place, and it was a very narrow lane of what was acceptable. I was big, I was black, and I was keenly aware of how I was treated because of it. It seemed I had nothing but white coaches telling me I was too stupid to play linebacker and black counselors telling me to stay away from white women— and nobody telling me to just go be whoever I wanted to be.

It was beyond frustrating because I *knew* that it was all a lie, I *knew* that racism was a Jedi mind trick. At the same time, I didn't yet know how to beat it or get around it. By my senior year, I was walking around going, "I hate all of this." It was the start of my militant phase, my Public Enemy phase. I was never as extreme as the guys walking around in dashikis and calling themselves Egyptian kings, but I did experience my first political awakening, crude as it was. I started looking at everything in racial terms. I saw *Do the Right Thing* in the theater probably twenty-five times. I'd never seen images so raw, so compelling, or so truthful. I wanted to write and direct my own movies, and Spike Lee was my hero. As *Star Wars* had done years earlier, *Do the Right Thing* cemented my conviction that I was meant to be in film someday.

I'm glad I went through that phase, because I think every young person needs to go through that phase of rebelling and questioning everything. But my militance wasn't a constructive militance, because it was driven by anger. Even when you have every right to be angry, anger is never helpful. It blinds you. That's what it did to me. On the football field, my anger became a form of self-sabotage. The smart thing to do would have been to be calculating about it: "Okay, these coaches are using me, so I'm going to use them right back to get what I want out of this deal. If I have to shovel shit to get what I want, then it is what it is." But I didn't do that. I didn't organize the players into a collective movement to stand up for better treatment, either. I just got pissed and started beefing with the coaches and getting in fights with the white players, all of which nearly torpedoed my chances in the NFL draft and didn't improve anything for me or anyone else.

What I wanted was something I couldn't find. I wanted that feeling I'd had at Interlochen the day of the competition, when the judge stood up and, because he was looking at my work and not at the color of my skin, chose my paintings as the best. Where could I go to get that feeling again? Where could I go to just be Terry Crews? I had no idea. Like my father, I was trapped between two Michigans, one foot in each, but belonging fully to neither. Being stuck in that trap had left my dad a lonely, angry, bitter alcoholic. So what was it going to do to me?

4

MALIBU'S MOST RACIST

After I started getting noticed with *Friday after Next*, I did a movie called *Malibu's Most Wanted*. It was one of the most heartbreaking, most racist experiences I've ever endured. In the movie, Jamie Kennedy, who was popular at the time, was playing a rich white kid from Malibu who's a wannabe gangster because he grew up watching nothing but BET and *Yo! MTV Raps*. Which is a problem for his dad, who's running for governor and wants his son to stop going around Malibu acting like a hood rat. He hires a couple of classically trained black actors to pretend to be thugs, kidnap the boy, and take him to the hood to see what real gangsters are like. Then he'll be scared into acting white again. But once the plan is put into action, the black guys pretending to be gangstas get kidnapped by black guys who are 100 percent real gangsters, and hilarity ensues.

Here I'll just point out that the film's director, its producers, and its writers were all rich and upper-middle-class white guys.

For a black person in a white world, there are so many obstacles to making it. First is having the awareness and the social connections to know how to get in and where to go to get work. Nobody told us that stuff back in Flint. I had to get "discovered" by a makeup artist while I was working as a security guard on a film set, hardly a traditional avenue into the business.

Second, even if you do manage to break in, there are few good opportunities for meaningful work. That's changing today, but back then, unless you landed a Spike Lee movie or a role on a "black" sitcom, the pickings were slim.

But one of the biggest challenges is that even when you're afforded the exact same opportunities as your white peers, your experience can be completely different. That had been true for me going all the way back to the NFL combine in Indianapolis my senior year of college. I was so excited showing up for that event. This was it, my pro football dream coming true. The reality was something else. We were all given T-shirts with a number. We put them on, and then we were paraded around in front of the scouts, like meat. As we walked, a man shouted "Take your shirts off," and we did so the scouts could see our muscle structure. "Turn to the front," he said. "Turn to the back." With every command, we did as we were told. Then they had a dentist come out and examine our teeth, like we were horses.

I couldn't help feeling that was the closest thing there is to a modern-day slave auction. The discomfort I felt was only compounded when I got to LA and discovered I now had an owner. In the NFL, you don't have a boss. You have an "owner," and your owner can keep you or trade you at their whim. That's hard-core. That's deep. That messes with your head. Of course, the white players had to stand up on the same auction block that I did. They signed a contract with their new "owners" as well. But that's exactly my point: even though we walked the same path, they weren't carrying nearly as much baggage. Maybe they didn't think twice about having an owner. I thought about it every damn day.

It was no different in Hollywood. My first big break, the reality show *Battle Dome*, was basically *American Gladiators* with a wrestling bent to it. In wrestling, everyone is a caricature. Everyone is a trope or a stereotype. There was the Superman guy and the goth rocker guy and the military guy wearing camouflage. But in America, it's a whole different experience being a black stereotype versus being a white ste- reotype. I played a gangster by the name of T- Money; my wife still calls me T-Money to this day. I was a warrior from the hood, from Detroit. I would cuss a lot and had a big gold chain with a dollar sign on it. I had a posse, and they would walk behind me wherever I went. Looking at it now, it's cringe-worthy times ten. But just like trying to get in the NFL, if you want the work and you want the opportunity, you suck it up and you do it.

Once I found my way to acting in comedies, life got exponentially more difficult. To be a black actor in the world of comedy is like tap-dancing blindfolded through a minefield. In any good comedy, you must be willing to be the butt of the joke. That's part of the deal. Everybody loves watching fools and buffoons get their comeuppance. That's been true since the time of Shakespeare. The baggage that black actors carry is two-hundred-plus years of popular entertain-ment that has mostly degraded black people and black culture as backward and ignorant. Nineteenth-century minstrel shows. Broad cartoonish stereotypes like Stepin Fetchit and Sleep n' Eat and Amos and Andy. It's hardly a distinguished legacy.

Jim Carrey and Ben Stiller and Will Ferrell have all built massive careers playing preening idiots who fall flat on their faces. Only when they do it, nobody accuses them of degrading and dehumanizing white people as a whole. Black actors, on the other hand, have to represent all black people at all times. Whenever you're playing a character who's the butt of the joke, with every beat of the story you have to ask yourself: Is the joke on my character or is it on my whole culture? Am I playing a clown, or being a coon? And, if this is the only work I'm being offered, how much choice do I have in the matter?

It's agonizing. And there's no avoiding it. Being able to laugh and poke fun at ourselves is a part of being human. It's cathartic. It's necessary. If black actors never played the fool, if we always had to be Denzel Washington as the noble warrior or Morgan Freeman as the wise old sage, that's dehumanizing, too. Because it doesn't show the full spectrum of what black life in the world is like.

So it's a problem, and *Malibu's Most Wanted* was a problem. Relative to most films of the time, it had several fairly substantial roles for black actors to play, by which I mean speaking parts with more than one line or one scene. Several talented and respected black actors signed on: Blair Underwood, Taye Diggs, Anthony Anderson, Regina Hall, Damien Wayans. I think we were all hoping the movie would be something better than what it was. There's a fine line between comedy that comments on and subverts racial stereotypes and comedy that exploits and reinforces them. *Malibu's Most Wanted* aspired to be the former, but far too often it ended up being the latter.

I played a tough guy named 8 Ball, who was part of Damien Wayans's crew. I did a lot of ad-libbing during the shooting, just goofing around with all these funny things on the set, dances and stuff. The director would always say, "Dude, that's funny. We're keeping that." I was loving it. I was living my Carol Burnett dream, making people laugh. The biggest moment in the movie for me was at the climax.

Jamie Kennedy was looking at his father, and they were having a big heart-to-heart talk. I didn't have a line, but as my character watched them hug and walk away arm in arm, I got all teary-eyed and said, "I wish I could talk to my pop like that. . . . I'm gonna call that nigga right now." Everyone cracked up because it came out of nowhere, and it was funny having this big, mean-looking dude having this emotional breakthrough. The director loved it and they decided to keep it.

Then, they called me back about a month later. Principal photography had ended. They were doing reshoots, and they had a joke that they wanted me to drop into the movie. I got to the set, and there was another black actor there. I hadn't met him before. He was an older guy, and he was even bigger than me. He was there to play my father in this scene they wanted to do. My only job was to stand there and look at this older guy while he said one line to me.

So I went and got on camera with the guy, and they yelled, "Action." He looked at me, and in this deep, booming voice, said, "Nigga . . . you will always be this nigga's nigga."

After the first take, I stood there frozen, like, "What's happening?" Over at the monitor, all these white writers and executives were cracking up, a couple of them with their hats turned backward and their Air Jordans on. I saw the guy who'd written the scene, and he was smiling big, like he was so proud. They were all like, "Do it again! Do it again!"

I didn't get it. The line I'd ad-libbed on set was an actual joke about the inability of fathers and sons to communicate (a subject I happened to know a thing or two about). This wasn't that. This was a bunch of white guys telling a couple of black actors to go all in on "nigga" with each other. And that wasn't even the end of it. We did it again, then we did it again, and then we did it again.

I felt bad enough just being a part of it. Then I saw Blair Underwood standing across the room. I caught his eye for a moment, and
he looked away as fast as he could. I knew exactly what he was thinking: "You're on your own for this one, Terry. I know you gotta do
what you gotta do, but *damn* . . ."

I felt awful. I felt dirty. And of course I didn't say anything. I was
too scared. I was a nobody trying to catch his big break. I had no
leverage to push back. Plus, I needed the paycheck.

I felt like I traded in a piece of myself on that one. It hurt. I let
these rich white guys do this to me because I didn't have the confidence to push back and say no or just walk off the set. I tried to blink
it away, but that eye contact with Blair seared the moment into my
brain: He had witnessed it, which meant I could never forget that it
had happened.

We finished up the scene and the director and producers said,
"That's a wrap, thank you!" I went home and I prayed and prayed
that the scene wouldn't make it into the movie. Thankfully, it didn't.
Somebody was looking out for me.

Nearly every black actor you meet in Hollywood has their *Malibu's Most Wanted* story. Probably several of them. People forget that
Morgan Freeman started out playing pimps before he became the
voice of God. Samuel L. Jackson has played more killers and murderers than he can remember. You feel it all the time in auditions, some
white casting director asking you, "Can you do it with, you know,
that walk? That thing?" They won't come right out and say "Be more
black," but that's what they mean.

Marvel used to call me in for auditions all the time. This was back
before *Black Panther* and Marvel started to turn things around. I'd
get called in for audition after audition, and I'd never get the roles
because they didn't actually call for a black actor. I remember going

in for the villain in the Hugh Jackman Wolverine movie *Logan*. The character was some redneck dude with a thick country accent. It was a part for a white guy, obviously. But I was there so that Marvel could check a box and fill a quota and say it auditioned a certain number of non-white actors for major roles before the directors went on and chose whatever white person they were planning on casting anyway. I finally asked my agent, "Why are you sending me in for all this stuff? This is a waste of my time."

He was like, "Well, do it anyway, because it might turn into something else."

Sometimes I would, and sometimes I wouldn't.

Talking to other black people in the business helped me a lot. One thing that was great about doing *Everybody Hates Chris* was that there were so many classic actors that came through. I got to act with Jimmie Walker and Debbie Allen, and with Ernest Lee Thomas from *What's Happening!!* Reggie Hudlin directed our pilot. They all had the same advice: You do what you have to do for your family and you make it work. You take the prisoner role or the gangster role and you do your best with them and, if you're lucky, you slowly amass the power not to have to do them anymore.

Ironically, the stuff that's obviously racist is in some ways the easiest to deal with. It is what it is. Either you're willing to put up with it for the paycheck or you're not. For me, what was harder to deal with were the situations where I felt stymied at every turn, but I didn't know if it was because of racism or not. That's the hardest question any black professional has to wrestle with: Is this harder for me because I'm black, or is it hard because it's hard?

I used to be afraid of walking the red carpet because it felt to me like the whitest thing ever. There were all those cameras and flashbulbs popping off. Maybe there would be a couple of black photographers in the mix, but in Hollywood it's a very white affair. The red carpet was hallowed ground, and I was always intimidated. I felt so, so small.

Every time I set foot on a red carpet, the same thing would happen. Some attractive young white lady would walk out, and all the photographers would scream her name and flip out and go crazy and take a thousand pictures. Then I would walk out after her and . . . crickets. Maybe one snap or two. They'd all but ignore me. Then I'd exit and the next white person would walk out and all the cameras would explode again.

I hated that feeling. I hated feeling insignificant just because I was standing next to a white person. I never wanted to go out and walk the red carpet. Rebecca had to push me. "Terry," she'd say, "this is your party. You did this project. You've got to take it and embrace it."

"Yeah," I'd say, "but these white people all think they're better than me."

"Terry, you've gotta do this because you're good enough and you have to know you're good enough."

I went home and started to recognize my feelings for what they were. Nobody was doing anything to me. The photographers want something that will sell, and their lazy assumption is that the photo of the white person who's already famous is going to sell better than the photo of the black guy who's famous mostly only to black people. But the reality is that the photo that's going to sell is whatever gets eyeballs and clicks. So I decided to give the photographers that. I started to do a thing on the red carpet where I would jump. I went out and announced it to the press. "Okay, guys, I'm gonna jump at the count of three and you're going to get me in midair." I did it, and they all got pictures of me, and the pictures sold. The next day the pictures were all over the papers and the movie blogs and the enter-tainment press.

Today, if you google "Terry Crews jumping," there are probably hundreds of pictures of me jumping in the air, because it became a thing. I'd come out and people would say, "Terry! Do the jump!" and I'd do the jump. There were white people next to me, and they were like, "Terry! Terry!" and the next day I'd be in the papers. And all the famous white people I'd resented for hogging the red carpet were loving it, too, calling my name and applauding for the jump and hav-ing fun with it and even standing back to give me room.

I realized, "Holy shit . . . I got it wrong." There I was, resenting "white people" for standing in the way of my success, when really it was me not understanding how the game was played and how I needed to play it. All of a sudden, all those feelings of resentment and insignificance left me. If I had never found the courage to deal with that and overcome it, those negative feelings would be festering to this day, with me sitting around and stewing about how I'll always be screwed because white people always win.

A similar thing happened on the set of *The Expendables*. There was so much hype surrounding that movie when it was announced because the cast was stacked with so many legends: Stallone, Schwar-zenegger, Bruce Willis, Dolph Lundgren, Jet Li, Jason Statham. The only reason my name made that list was because Wesley Snipes was in jail on his tax thing. Stallone had called me in at the last minute because I had the muscles for it.

My first few weeks on set were pretty miserable. I went in with low expectations simply because my character's name was originally going to be Jazz Gumbo. I read that and said, "Oh, I guess I know what this is going to be." Luckily they changed it to Hale Caesar. Still, name change or no, for the first few weeks I sat in my hotel room. They weren't using me for anything. All the major action was going to the boldfaced names and my character was getting shunted so far to the background I felt like I was practically part of the scenery. Same as with the red carpet photos. I would sit in my trailer and stew about how racist Hollywood was and how it never respected me and how the only reason I was on that set was to be the token black guy. I told myself, "I'm going to say my lines and get out of here. I'm gonna mail it in. Whatever."

Then I caught myself. I remembered the red carpet. I remembered what had come from giving my all to sweeping floors at Labor Ready and always pressing my shirts to work security on film sets. A positive attitude had flipped both of those things to my advantage. So I turned my mind around. I said to myself, "Terry, man, listen. You are becoming cynical. You have to give it your all. Maybe this is racism and maybe it's not, but you won't know unless you give it your all. If you take yourself out while you're in the middle of this, you're guaranteed nothing. You need to straighten your attitude out and be a professional, no matter what, and let the universe handle the rest."

I started showing up on set and throwing myself into every scene. I was talking to everyone, meeting everyone, just giving off positive vibes and energy every minute of the day. Stallone and I went from being complete strangers who barely spoke to each other on set to talking through scenes together every single day. When Rebecca came to visit the set, Stallone was talking to her and he said, "Your husband is rocking every scene. I'm rewriting the script so that he saves all of our lives at the end. I'm rewriting everything to highlight him." Lo and behold, that's what ended up being the big climax of the movie. Stallone wrote a big scene where I come through the tunnel and blow all the bad guys up and save them. That was all changed in the last two weeks of shooting, purely because of the attitude I brought to the set.

I'm not saying that a positive mental attitude and an upbeat personality will get a Klansman to put down his torch and give you a
hug. A positive mental attitude would not have salvaged *Malibu's
Most Wanted* from being what it was. But what I am saying is that
most social or workplace interactions are far more nuanced than
what happened to me on *Malibu's Most Wanted*. Every situation car-
ries with it the potential for social miscues and misunderstanding. If
you go into those interactions expecting the worst, you're going to
get it. Because all you get back from any situation is what you put
into it. If you go in expecting everyone to be racist, like I initially did
with *The Expendables*, then you're not going to connect with anyone
on any genuine level. The conversations will be stilted, everyone's
body language will be cold, and the lack of connection will only further your belief that everyone around you is, in fact, racist. It becomes a self-fulfilling prophecy. However, if you go in putting out
nothing but positive vibes, if you start from the default position that
everyone is trying their best and any miscommunication or ignorant
comment is just that, then you neutralize a lot of awkwardness before it ever comes to the surface. More important, you've forged genuine relationships and friendships that will help you work through
any problems that do arise.

And I don't say that to minimize the amount of racism in Hollywood. Not at all. In fact, my point is this: Given the large amount of
racism that does exist in Hollywood, it doesn't serve me to go looking
for it when it isn't there. Now, anytime I hit a wall, I take the default
assumption that the situation is hard because it's hard, not hard
because I'm black. And when I do encounter racism, I never have to
sit around wondering, "Is this racist?" The racism makes itself plain,
and unlike when I was working on *Malibu's Most Wanted*, I've learned
how to deal with it.

Not too long after I started doing the red carpet jump, right around the time I filmed the pilot for *Brooklyn Nine-Nine*, Adam Sandler called me. We'd done *The Longest Yard* together, and he had another part he wanted me to do. It was him and his whole usual gang and they were making a movie in South Africa, *Blended*, about a single dad and a single mom who end up stuck together on vacation in Africa. They hate each other but then of course they end up falling for each other. He sent me the script and I read it and . . . my jaw was on the floor. The romantic comedy part of the movie was fine, but the character he was asking me to play was one of the most offensive things I'd ever read in a Hollywood movie script . . . and that's saying something.

The character that had been written is an entertainer at a big South African resort. It's a scene where he's supposed to be entertaining a dinner crowd. He comes out into the dining room in a grass skirt with a spear and his face painted. Then he starts running around scaring the dinner guests, going, "Ooga booga! Ooga booga! ARGGHH!!!" Then he gets up onstage and says, in this posh British accent, "Hello! My name is Nickens!"

I wish I were making this up. It was horrible. It was extremely degrading to African people. This shit would have been racist in 1913, and we were in 2013. And this movie had been green-lighted by Warner Bros. Everybody had read the script and signed off. They were in preproduction. Serious money was being spent to make this.

I called my manager and said, "I can't do this."

"Oh my god, I know," he said. "I just read it, too. I couldn't believe it."

First of all, I couldn't believe the movie was even being made with this scene in it. Second of all, it's not like I was some random actor at that point. Adam Sandler wasn't my best friend, but we were really cool with each other. We'd worked together and always had great times. I couldn't believe that he'd actually sent this to me thinking I would do it. Still, the fact that he and I were friendly told me one important thing: he wasn't trying to be racist. He actually, honestly, didn't know how offensive this thing was. So I said to my manager, "Let me call Adam and talk to him."

Then I did something I'd never done in Hollywood before. I spoke up. I'd passed on parts before, declined things I didn't want to participate in. But I'd never spoken up. You learn pretty quickly not to complain in the entertainment business, about racism or anything else. Because the default mentality is "Shut up and do the thing we're telling you to do, and if you won't, we'll find somebody who will." And they can, because they'll never run out of people desperate enough to do it. But I'd just been through the whole D-Day aftermath with Rebecca, going to therapy and learning how to handle things better, and for the first time in my career I felt like I had the leverage to say something.

I also felt like Adam might be open to talking because of what we'd been through on *The Longest Yard*. We'd had some hard-core moments doing that. Lots of big black dudes playing prisoners, lots of big white guys playing prison guards, and it got heated. There were moments when the guards were screaming at us, going, "I'm gonna make you my bitch, nigger," and all the black people on the set felt like, "Uh, these dudes ain't acting." There were also some fight scenes that got out of hand, beyond what was supposed to happen in the script, and I felt Adam was at least aware enough to know he didn't want things to go wrong like that again. So I called him.

"Bro," I said, "you've gotta understand, if I did this, black people would never talk to me again, and it wouldn't be too pleasant for you, either."

For a minute or two, he still didn't get it. He was like, "Whaddya mean? You don't think it's funny?"

"Adam. *Dude*. It's really, really bad. It's not going to work."

Then I made a suggestion. I said, "I can't do this the way it is, but why don't you let me try to redo it in a way that I feel would actually be great? And if you don't like it, I understand."

And Adam, to his credit, said, "All right, I'll see what you got."

So now I was back to the problem of how to play the fool as a black man in America. How was I going to Will Ferrell this thing to make the character ridiculous but in a way that didn't read as degrading to black people in general and South African people in particular?

I sat on it, and the idea I came up with was to make him sort of an African Wayne Newton, all the preening ridiculousness of a Las Vegas showman, but transplanted to an African resort. Now it was about an individual being self-centered and narcissistic as opposed to lampooning the culture of an entire continent with a spear and a grass skirt. I spent five grand and got a wig made and then I spent another five grand and had all these African suits done. We got Ladysmith Black Mambazo, the famous South African group, to back me up as my band, and we worked on songs together and the songs were catchy and authentic to the place where we were filming.

And we stole the movie. It was hilarious. The writers loved it and they kept calling me back to set and adding new scenes for me. When we wrapped the film Adam told me, "Dude, I'm so glad that you came up with all of this. This is way better than what we had in the script." And I thanked him. I thanked him for listening because most people in Hollywood wouldn't have been open to changing it, and if we hadn't changed it, it would have been a disaster.

Blended is not the greatest movie ever made. It's not even the best Adam Sandler movie ever made. But it's one of the most important films in my career because it's the movie where I finally did what I should have done but was too scared to do on *Malibu's Most Wanted*. I turned around, faced the problem, talked to the powers that be, and found a way to a solution that worked for everyone.

5

TRUE POWER

I n July 2013, I was on the set of *Brooklyn Nine-Nine*, shooting one of the episodes from our first season. We were in between scenes, and I was sitting at my desk checking my phone when the news hit Twitter. George Zimmerman had been acquitted for the killing of Trayvon Martin in Sanford, Florida. I couldn't believe it. Zimmerman, who was not a police officer, had followed a young black teenager around his own neighborhood, and baited him into a fight. Then, when that child ended up dead by a bullet from Zimmerman's gun, the man claimed self-defense and a jury let him walk? I was disgusted and appalled.

Then I started reading past the headline and into people's comments. I was even more disgusted and appalled. Zimmerman's supporters were outside courthouse waving signs that read SELF-DEFENSE IS A BASIC HUMAN RIGHT. People were calling Trayvon a thug, saying he deserved it, and worse. But the most disturbing thing I read was the reports of people cheering when the verdict came through.

People were driving around, honking their horns, acting like their team had won a big game. That was confounding, because *even if* you believed Zimmerman's bogus claim of self-defense, *even if* you thought his actions were somehow justified, that didn't change the fact that a child was dead. There was nothing to celebrate.

I was shocked, but I shouldn't have been surprised, because it was a thing I'd witnessed once before. In 1995, my journeyman football career had taken me to Washington, DC, and I was already getting burned out on the game. My eyes were turning more and more toward the world of entertainment, and in those days, DC was still the headquarters for BET, Black Entertainment Television. If you were black and wanted to be in show business back then, BET was the mother ship, so I finagled some connections through the NFL to get a meeting at the network, thinking Rebecca and I might get involved there somehow.

On the morning of October 3, we drove in together for the meeting. Once we were done, before heading home to Virginia, we stopped to grab a bite in the BET cafeteria. It just so happened that while we were sitting there, up on the TV screen, the verdict was about to be read in the trial of O. J. Simpson for the murder of his ex-wife Nicole Brown Simpson and her boyfriend Ronald Goldman. For months the case had been on everyone's minds, and while it was obvious to anyone following along that O. J. was guilty, it was also true that the LAPD had its own crimes to account for.

Having lived in Los Angeles as a big black guy, I knew all about the LAPD. The most harrowing run-in I had with them happened when I first arrived to play with the Rams. It was right in the wake of the LA riots. The LAPD officers who'd beaten Rodney King had all been acquitted, the city had exploded with pent-up frustration and rage, and Reginald Denny had been dragged from his truck and assaulted. In the middle of the afternoon, I was driving on the 101 in

my Nissan Pathfinder. I got pulled over, and four cops from two pa-
trol cars came at me with guns drawn, shouting at me through a
megaphone to roll the windows down and put my hands where they
could see them. Because I can't hear very well, I have a hard time
understanding people when I can't see their lips. I was petrified I
might mishear what they were telling me and end up getting shot. I
sat in the driver's seat like a statue, the red and blue lights flashing,
all four windows down, my hands glued to the steering wheel. It was
the most frightening thing I've ever experienced, and it's hard to
describe, the feeling of knowing that with one wrong move your life
could be over. It's so intense it's like you're outside of yourself watching yourself go through it.

And the reason they'd pulled me over? The tint on my car windows was too dark. The kept me there on the side of the freeway for
an hour and a half, and pretty soon it was rush hour and the road
was packed and all the drivers were rubbernecking from the cars
going past, which made the whole thing degrading as well as terrifying.

The problem wasn't just in LA, either. A couple of years later, after
I got cut from the Packers and signed at the last minute by the Chargers, I had to jump on a plane to San Diego with literally a few hours'
notice. I paid cash for my ticket when I boarded in Kalamazoo, and
when we landed for a connection in Chicago, a bunch of armed police
boarded the plane and pulled me straight out of my seat. They were
real aggressive, too, talking to me like cops on TV. "You. Over here.
Now."

Once I was off the plane, they had me up against the wall of the
gangway, their hands on their guns as they grilled me. "What's the
nature of your business on this flight?"

"I'm going to San Diego."

"Why are you going to San Diego?"

We kept going back and forth and, it turns out, they thought I was a drug dealer because I'd paid cash for my ticket.

"Officer," I said, staying as calm as I could. "I'm a professional football player. I've just been picked up by the San Diego Chargers and I paid cash because it was a last-minute flight."

"Ohhhhh . . ." they said, suddenly all apologetic.

Then they asked for my autograph.

It was the weirdest, most offensive thing ever. But as pissed off as I was, I signed every last one, forcing a smile on my face to make sure the TV cop routine didn't start up again. When I got back on the plane, all the other passengers were staring at me. But I didn't care. I was just happy I hadn't been arrested or shot.

Getting let off the hook for being an NFL player was my first experience with the benefits of what would later become recognition and fame. I can't count the number of times I've had police officers approach me because of my size and my skin color, only to visibly relax and take their hands off their sidearms once they realize that they've seen me on TV before. I've often wondered, especially given my problems with anger and rage, what might have happened to me if I hadn't become famous, if I'd remained just another big black guy.

Sitting in the BET cafeteria that day, I was a long way from being famous. Like everyone else, I was just somebody on pins and needles to see what the outcome of the trial would be. As we waited for the decision, the cafeteria started filling up. People kept streaming in to huddle around the television, and pretty soon it was packed with people. Then the verdict finally came back: not guilty. The whole room erupted in cheers. People where whooping and hollering and cheering. They were throwing things. They were cheering like the Bullets had just won the NBA championship.

Rebecca and I sat there in silence, horrified. Having been humiliated by the cops as often as I have, I understood the desire to get some payback. Still, sitting there in the cafeteria, all I could think was "Okay. But two people are dead. Nicole Brown Simpson and Ronald Goldman are dead. The Browns and the Goldmans have each lost a child. O. J.'s children have lost their mother. This is a tragedy." Even if you thought O. J. was innocent—and, trust me, *nobody* in that room thought O. J. was innocent—there was nothing to rejoice about in any of it, just like there was nothing to rejoice in the death of Trayvon Martin. Yet all around me, people were ecstatic, celebrating the murder of two innocent people. It was one of the most vile things I've ever witnessed in my life, and it was my own people doing it.

Ever since that day at Interlochen when my paintings were judged solely on their merit, my life has been one nonstop journey to find what I felt that day: a place where I can define my own identity and be seen simply as myself. At times that journey has felt more like a war, and it's always been a war being fought on two fronts. Even as I've struggled with the bigotry of racist cops and the stereotypes of the Hollywood machine, I've also had to wrestle with the hatred, closed-mindedness, and intolerance that come from my own community. It's been happening ever since I can remember. Back in Flint, it was the black counselor who told me to "stay away from white women" and all the black kids in the street who physically threatened me for going to an integrated school and being "too white." In college, it was the militant black studies crowd who rejected me simply because I couldn't go along with their us-versus-them mentality. Since then it's mostly been because of my marriage, because of my "white wife."

My wife is black. Her father may be white. She may look white. But her mother is black, and her mother gave birth to her in Gary, Indiana, in 1965, when the one-drop rule was still in full effect. Also, anyone who knows this country's history of slavery and rape and white men forcing themselves on black women knows full well that "black people" can come out looking all sorts of different ways. (I'm 15 percent Scotch-Irish myself—don't know where, don't know how—but you'd never know to look at me.) My wife grew up a black woman in a black household in a black neighborhood, suffused with black culture. But none of that has stopped the dirty looks she gets pretty much everywhere she goes.

When she was named Miss Gary 1984, a lot of black people resented her and hated her for it, as if it were only because she had some kind of magic ticket or some extra favor. Folks would get in her face and say, "It's just because you're part white." She'd have to say, "Well, I can't do anything about that. I'm just here. I don't know what else to tell you."

One of the most painful rejections came when we first tried to find a church after moving to Los Angeles. Faithful Central is a black church in Inglewood. We went there and sat in the back for a few weeks to check it out. I didn't care much either way, but Rebecca fell in love. "This is such a wonderful place," she said, looking at all the nice families and the kids running around. "We're going to join."

So one Sunday at the end of the service, we went up to the altar to formally join the church. The second we stepped up, we could hear audible gasps and whispers behind us. I couldn't help but turn around to see all these black women with daggers coming out of their eyes. They were crossing their arms, scowling at me, doing everything they could to let me know we were not welcome.

We turned back to the altar, shook the pastor's hand, and went back to our seats. Then, as we were walking out to our car, I said, "Becky, did you see that?"

"Yeah," she said. "I saw it. We can't go back."

And we never did. Which is how we ended up at Faith Community out in West Covina, because the mostly Hispanic congregation we met there had no problem with us.

And that's never changed. When we did our BET reality show, *The Family Crews*, my oldest daughters, who are very fair skinned, got tons of hate mail. I'm talking about grown black people sending hate mail to black children. When I started doing *Everybody Hates Chris* and *Brooklyn Nine-Nine* I was nominated several years running for the NAACP Image Awards. Rebecca came with me. Walking down the red carpet, we would get the same cutting, evil looks we'd seen at church, all these black women rolling their eyes and going, "Mmmmmm-hmmmmm." As of now, we've just stopped going.

In 2016, ESPN released *O.J.: Made in America*, a five-part documentary that digs deep into the history and racial politics behind the O. J. Simpson trial, and one of the most fascinating aspects of it is the way it covers the jury selection. There were eight black women on the twelve-person jury. The prosecutor, Marcia Clark, a white woman, had pushed to get those black women on the jury, thinking their sympathies would lie with O. J.'s battered and murdered wife. But Johnnie Cochran, the lone black attorney on O. J.'s defense team, knew better. He wanted those same black women on the jury because he knew what Clark did not. He knew those black women would be looking for payback against not just the LAPD. He also knew that those black women would look at Nicole Brown Simpson the same way they look at my wife, with zero empathy. A juror who was interviewed basically came right out and said as much. Even with everything I've seen Rebecca endure, I was still shocked by the callousness of the statement when I heard it.

Being so twisted up in your own hate that it's left you indifferent to murder . . . I don't even have the words for it. It's a whole other level of evil. I don't care if you're cheering George Zimmerman for killing Trayvon Martin or cheering O. J. Simpson for killing Nicole Brown Simpson and Ronald Goldman. Both of those things are evil. Even with all the harm that white America has visited upon black

America over the centuries, I fail to see how you can make a moral distinction between the two.

I am often told that "only white people can be racist." That idea has always struck me as a semantic argument that hinges on a very narrow, very American definition of "racist," given that people of every color, ethnicity, and creed have been conquering, subjugating, and killing each other all over the globe for millennia. Still, even if you accept the premise that only white people can be racist, no group of people is unique in its capacity for evil. No matter how right our cause or how just our motivation, we are all human and therefore fallible. Indeed, it is often in the moment where we feel the zeal of righteousness and justice the most that we are at the greatest risk of succumbing to our own worst impulses.

IN THE LATE SPRING OF 2020, like the rest of America, I was hunkered down at home in quarantine, trying to get through early months of the COVID pandemic. Lockdown had been a particularly trying time for us because of Rebecca's condition: just two weeks before the shutdown began, she'd had a double mastectomy. Seeing her in the hospital after the surgery was a gut-wrenching experience, because it was first time that I had ever realized that I might be without her. After thirty-two years together, I don't know where I begin and she ends anymore. We're simply a part of each other, and the thought that I might lose her was incredibly scary. Once we got home, she was weak and couldn't move around much. I did my best to stay busy nursing her back to health, changing her bandages and making her meals, doing what I could to push the fear and the worry to the back of my mind. But then, once the lockdown started and the whole world skidded to a halt, it was just me and her and our son, alone in the silence.

Those first months of the pandemic were a strange time, one in which the best way to "do something" was to stay home and do nothing. When that isolation and uncertainty landed on top of Rebecca's recovery, it put me in this mindset of "You have to stay strong, Terry. You can't break. You have to be here for her. You have to be her rock. In this crisis, you have to be the kind of man she'd be proud of. You have to be ready to take on the whole world because she can't do it on her own right now."

As the lockdown entered its third month, on May 26, after finishing up a Zoom interview with *The View* to promote the season fifteen premiere of *America's Got Talent*, I clicked over to surf the web. With reality on lockdown, the internet—and social media in particular— had become my reality. It seems like that was true for all of us. Practically every hour on the hour, I would surf the web, looking for updates on when the lockdown would be over. That's what I was doing when I came across a *New York Times* article about the death of yet another unarmed black man in police custody.

The headline read BYSTANDER VIDEOS OF GEORGE FLOYD AND OTHERS ARE POLICING THE POLICE. The article itself went on to highlight the discrepancies between the police report and actual cell phone footage of the man's death by the incident's bystanders. The police had claimed that Floyd had died on his way to the hospital; the videos told a different, more accurate, story. I read the article. I didn't watch the video. As more and more of those videos have gone viral in recent years, I've made a practice of avoiding them. While I understand the necessity of people seeing them, I usually can't bring myself to do it. This time, however, it seemed there was no escaping it. The video followed me onto Twitter and then onto TikTok, popping up everywhere I went, and I finally relented and clicked play.

What I saw shocked me to my core. A police officer kneeling with his full weight on George Floyd's neck as he moaned and cried out, "I can't breathe." Bystanders were pleading with the officer to let him up, but the officer just stayed there until the man eventually grew quiet. When it was over, it hit me that I'd just watched a man die—a big, black man who looked a lot like me. George Floyd was, at that point, the newest in a long and growing list of names with which America had become all too familiar: Michael Brown, Tamir Rice, Freddie Gray, Eric Garner, Philando Castile, Sandra Bland, Alton Sterling, Breonna Taylor. Tension and anger were building.

In that moment, I felt the same way I'd felt sitting on the set of *Brooklyn Nine-Nine* reading all the Harvey Weinstein stories: I felt I needed to say something. I went over to my Instagram page and shared some of my own experiences of being on the business end of a jumpy police officer's gun. "I could have been George Floyd," I said, hoping to help people understand how common these police encounters are. The reaction was beyond supportive. Don Lemon had me on CNN to discuss what I'd said, and it felt like the whole world was nodding along, understanding what I and thousands of others were going online to say.

As the video of Floyd's death continued to go viral, the outpouring of public opinion remained overwhelmingly positive. The vast majority of people pouring into the streets and posting online merely wanted to pay tribute to the man who'd been killed, see that justice was done for the crime, and see reforms put in place to make sure that this tragedy stops unfolding again and again. All of which was wonderful to see.

All the same, I couldn't help but feel a darker element starting to rise, like a weed growing among flowers, a disturbing undertow in the tidal wave of emotion that was sweeping over the country. It wasn't any one tweet or any one Facebook post that set me off, just the general tone of so much of the discourse. People had every right to be angry, but this was a different kind of rage. What I saw was a broad-brush, categorical demonization and dehumanization of "white people." It was "white people" this and "white people" that. Phrases like "white supremacy" and "white privilege" were being thrown around in ways far beyond their intended definitions, making it sound as if "whiteness" were some kind of original sin, an inherent defect that made every white person complicit in Floyd's murder. It made me feel, quite honestly, like I was back in the BET cafeteria, where black people were so angry, so eager for payback, that they lost all perspective on what was right and just and humane.

All the sweeping generalizations about "white people" disturbed me. First of all, I knew that they just weren't true. Second of all, once you start demonizing "white people" and "whiteness," you're setting yourself up as judge and jury of any black person you deem to be "too white" and therefore "insufficiently black." I've been down that road. It's where black people run my wife out of church and send hate mail to my children. It's not a good place to be.

But even more important than that is the fact that dehumanizing white people is dehumanizing to black people. The first step in losing our own humanity is dehumanizing others, because it's the justification we use to trespass against them. In order to maintain the slave economy of the South, America had to convince itself that black people were less than human. They cultivated a whole mythology about the black man's "base instincts" and "animal nature" in order to justify keeping millions of people in bondage. By creating and investing themselves in that mythology, by failing to recognize the humanity of black people, the white slaveholders of the South turned themselves into moral monsters.

The opposite of dehumanization is empathy, recognition. Anytime we recognize and empathize with the humanity of the person sitting across from us, we're less likely to use our power to inflict harm on them. But the moment we start to see them as different from and less than us, the door is open for us to commit any manner of crime against them, from everyday disrespect up to and including lynching and genocide. By dehumanizing others, we start to lose our own moral compass, our own goodness, and thus our own humanity.

I know it's true because I'm a textbook example. Being a toxic male chauvinist addicted to pornography, I saw my wife and other women as objects, which gave rise to my controlling, abusive temper. As the child of an abusive home, for a long time I saw Big Terry not as the broken, damaged person he was, but as an evil monster to be defeated, which ended up with my beating my own father bloody at Christmas, one of the lowest, rock-bottom points of my life. I've had to learn how to have empathy, and it's hard. I have to practice at it every day, and I still fail all the time.

Sitting in my house under lockdown, looking out on the world through the distorted lens of Twitter and Instagram, I felt like our empathy for each other was slipping away. What was especially disturbing was the heightening effect that social media was having. When I was in college, the same toxic elements of black militance were already there—the demonization of white people as "blue-eyed devils" and the ridiculous notions of melanin making black people superior somehow. But those ideas could only go so far outside the bubble of the black fraternity. You couldn't just sit around and marinate in hating white people all the time. You were an extreme minority on campus. At the end of the day, you had to go out and interact with white professors and white classmates and, as much as some of them might piss you off, you had to learn how to get along and empathize and relate to others.

A lot of the militance was performative as well. You had to do it for the group so that no one would come down on you for not supporting the cause. Guys would put on the black beret and the dashiki and shout, "Man, *fuck* white people." But then once the show was over they'd drop the act and go home to their white friends and white girlfriends and, in some cases, their white family members. You could be as militant as you wanted—and I went through that phase as well—but at some point you had to reconcile your ideology with the demands of reality.

Now, thanks to social media, when people are online, they never have to leave their bubbles, and everyone is performing all the time— a phenomenon exacerbated by the isolation brought on by the pandemic. On Facebook and Twitter, people live in these echo chambers where they not only can never drop the act, but have to constantly dial up the volume to prove their bona fides to anyone who is watching— and *everyone* is watching. Every private thought has become a public utterance. As that has happened, the nuance and ambivalence of private reflection and interpersonal dialogue has vanished from the conversation. Every statement has become more strident, more militant, more judgmental, and more vicious.

I understood what was happening on a visceral level because I'd grown up in it. The screaming mobs on Twitter reminded me of the congregation at Greater Holy Temple Church of God in Christ, whipped up into a self-righteous frenzy by Elder Jones. In that church, everybody was watching everybody, passing judgment on every sin and denouncing all the heathen non-believers outside who were surely going to hell. My mother passed judgement on everyone for their sins because she was so afraid that she'd get caught out for her own. Being holier than thou was the smokescreen that kept other people from opening her closet door and finding all those Harlequin romance novels inside. Now, that same dynamic was playing out in the digital public square 24/7, replicating all the worst aspects of being trapped inside a cult.

Any culture can become a cult, no matter how pure and noble its intentions. The words of Jesus Christ contain not one passage about being judgmental and cruel to your fellow man. In fact, everything He said was the opposite. Yet the Greater Holy Temple Church of God in Christ exists, sowing judgment and cruelty in Jesus's name. It's a phenomenon that transcends any one ideology. From Donald Trump's MAGA hordes to Bernie Sanders's Bernie Bros to the fanboys of the Marvel Cinematic Universe—every group is out there in their Twitter bubble, led by their loudest and angriest adherents. Everyone in the bubble who Likes and retweets the popular prevailing sentiment gets showered with Likes and retweets of their own. Anyone who pushes back against that sentiment invites a torrent of verbal abuse. By gifts we make slaves, and by whips we make dogs. There's nothing new under the sun.

Social media makes people cruel in the same way that religion made my mother cruel. It made her self-righteous. She was so convinced of the rightness of her actions—or, more precisely, she so desperately needed to *convince herself* of the rightness of her actions—that she decided she was justified in abusing others who couldn't or wouldn't follow the same rules. The same thing was true of me for a long time, because in my shame I'd learned to be just as judgmental and self-righteous as she was. Once I understood that, I came to realize that self-righteousness is perhaps the greatest sin of all, because it's yet another justification we give ourselves to excuse the damage we inflict.

Self-righteousness is the thing that allows us to lift ourselves up in the same way that dehumanizing others allows us to lower them down. Once we allow that dynamic to take root, we've created a moral monster—and the monster is ourselves. Maybe it's true that "only white people can be racist," but anyone can fall into the trap of dehumanizing others. Anyone can become so convinced of the goodness of their cause that they will excuse any action that supports it, and in the end they will wind up no better than the abusers they set out to destroy.

All of which is to say that in the wake of George Floyd's murder, I was witnessing a number of disturbing trends that had started to bubble up online. This movement to save black lives, born of the best intentions—intentions with which I fully agree—appeared to me to be curdling into something else. After watching this unhealthy dynamic play out for the week and a half after Floyd's murder, I decided I ought to say something. There were plenty of racist trolls flaming black people right back, but it didn't seem like people were stepping in to try to bring the dialogue back to a constructive place. So I decided to give it a shot. After all, it had worked before. When I jumped on Twitter and shared my thoughts and experiences in support of the Me Too movement, it had ended with victory against William Morris and my testifying before Congress. What could go wrong? So on June 7, I tweeted out:

> Defeating White Supremacy without White people
> creates Black Supremacy. Equality is the truth. Like it
> or not, we are all in this together.

I posted the tweet, went out to pick up some fast food for lunch with my son, and when I got back to my computer, it was like I'd set the internet on fire. The phrase "Black Supremacy" was the fuse on a powder keg. It was the number one trending topic on all of Twitter.

When I'd first tweeted out the phrase "Black Supremacy," I did it because it just came to me as the most succinct way of expressing what I was thinking, a way to take the pervasive anti-white bigoted attitudes I'd encountered my whole life and sum them up while staying within Twitter's limited word count; I wasn't even aware of any other contexts in which it had been used. Then, once the backlash hit, I started digging and found, of course, that I was far from the only person to use it.

"Black supremacy," Martin Luther King Jr. said in 1960, "is as dangerous as white supremacy, and God is not interested merely in the freedom of black men and brown men and yellow men. God is interested in the freedom of the whole human race and in the creation of a society where all men can live together as brothers, where every man will respect the dignity and the worth of human personality." Which is pretty much exactly what I'd meant to say; it's no surprise that Dr. King said it more eloquently than I had.

It was also no surprise that the backlash came swift and hard. I received both public and private messages that I should rescind the statement or I would be rescinded. People called me an Uncle Tom. My feed was filling up with pictures of clowns and coons. One prominent black performer accused me of being "an enemy of the people." Another said my tweet was a "capitulation to White Supremacy."

Part of the reason it's easy to get sucked into a Twitter beef is that you end up taking a ton of incoming fire, and so much of it is so off the mark you feel that you *have* to respond. In the messages I was receiving, I was being told, over and over, that black supremacy could never be a problem because black people are only 13 percent of the US population and we hold "no institutional power." First of all, as Dr. King knew, any kind of supremacy is a belief system. It's not about how much power you have in the moment. It's about the reasons you have for seeking power and what you would do with power if you got it. Are you out there marching for George Floyd because you want to reconcile and unite everyone in a country built on dignity and respect and equality? Or are you out there filled with self-righteous rage because you believe, deep down, that white people are morally defective and non-white people are in some way superior?

As to the point that black people have "no institutional power," that's just not true, and it's astonishing to me that someone would make that claim. Fifty years after Stokely Carmichael raised his fist on a march in Mississippi, defiantly calling on black people to assert their power, why would black people try to rally themselves, disclaiming the considerable power that we already have? Do black people have as much power as white people? Of course not. We're a small minority of the population. Do black people have as much power as we *should*? Of course not. The legacy of slavery and segregation has left us with vast disparities that remain to be overcome. But over the last ten to fifteen years, black people elected a black president. Black voters in South Carolina single-handedly determined the course of the 2020 Democratic primary, making Joe Biden the party's nominee. Despite the wealth gap that persists, black households generate billions of dollars in personal income every year. Every university and Fortune 500 company in America is out there tap-dancing as fast as it can to prove how "diverse" it can be. Why? Because we have power. We have political power, economic power, and cultural power—and as history has shown, time and again, any group of people is just as capable of abusing its power as anyone else. Black people can use our power responsibly to pursue justice for ourselves and reconciliation for all, or we can abuse it in ways that dehumanize others and further divide the country.

And yet, for some reason, the world still insists on seeing black people as powerless. When this whole back and forth was going on, I was getting tweets, not just from black people but also from white people, all these eighteen- and nineteen-year-old super-woke white kids telling me how powerless I am, that I am a victim of white supremacy, that I need to "do the work" so I can understand the ways in which "whiteness" is "controlling" me.

But it's not.

It used to, certainly. For the longest time I was controlled, not just by racism but by my rage and my shame and everything else. I saw myself as nothing but a victim, coming and going. I was a victim of my parents' abuse, a victim of my coaches' abuse, a victim of all the white directors and producers who wanted to cast me as only criminals and gangsters. I could blame everyone else for every problem in my life, and I did. I could luxuriate in victimhood forever, and I did. There were days it felt as good as a warm bubble bath. But then comes the downside of it, because seeing yourself as a victim means you see yourself as powerless, and the impotence of being powerless leaves you with nothing but rage. I understood that rage all too well. I lived with it for most of my life, which is why I recognized it in so many of the voices I saw crying out on Twitter in the wake of George Floyd.

My understanding of the power that I have started to change only after D-Day with Rebecca, but it finally, completely turned around thanks to Adam Venit. For the year I spent sitting around, frustrated, watching my work opportunities dry up and waiting for William Morris to do something, I was 100 percent the victim in the situation. Then, inspired by the courage of the women who stood up to Harvey Weinstein, once I went public about my assault, I never once felt like a victim again. Even sitting across from Ari Emanuel, even being threatened by one of the most powerful men in Hollywood, I never saw myself as powerless. "No, no, no," I said. "I'm the one driving this train. I have the power here. I am the one in control of how I handle this situation."

And because I decided to be, I was.

The same thing was true in the wake of George Floyd's murder. In that moment, black people wielded a *tremendous* amount of power. The eyes of the whole world were upon us. Our words were the top-trending subjects on every social media platform in the country.

Books about race were flying off the shelves and filling up virtually every last slot on the *New York Times* bestseller list. We were given a gigantic megaphone, so it was important that we stopped and asked ourselves, "What do we want to say?"

As Viktor Frankl wrote, in that moment, we were in control of how we used our power to respond to a gross injustice. Would we abuse that power, or would we use it responsibly in a way that moved the country forward and not back? Every few minutes, I was getting another tweet that indicated the former and not the latter. The one response that really said it all was from a black writer for *The Root* and other publications. She said, "You truly are worthless to us. White people can have you, especially since you love doing their work for them." It was the kind of response that only proved everything I was saying was right. We were in danger of destroying a potential moment of unity, reconciliation, and progress by turning it into a bitter, zero-sum game of black against white—and here this woman's reply boiled the issue down to exactly that: If you're not with "us," you're with "them."

Upstairs in the bedroom, Rebecca was following along on her phone. I asked her what she thought I should do, and she was in the same place I was. She's experienced the bigotry of black people, even more than I have, and after facing her own mortality just a few weeks before, she didn't have time for anything other than blunt honesty and truth. "Terry," she said, "do not back down. You're doing a good thing." So I didn't back down. The next day I followed my "Black Supremacy" tweet with this one:

> Please know that everything I've said comes from
> a spirit of love and reconciliation, for the Black
> community first, then the world as a whole, in hopes
> to see a better future for Black people. I believe it
> is important we not suffer from groupthink, and

we keep minds of our own, and be allowed to
ask difficult questions to each other. I believe this
dialogue is important as we get through this trauma
together. I love you.

And I followed that one with:

If you are a child of God, you are my brother and
sister. I have family of every race, creed and ideology.
We must ensure #blacklivesmatter doesn't morph
into #blacklivesbetter

Of course, #blacklivesbetter lit an even bigger powder keg than
"Black Supremacy" had, and from there the backlash only continued. The clown and coon images kept flooding in. The rapper Rick
Ross even put a line about me into one of his singles, saying "Terry
Crews is a coon who was basically bought." This from a man who
raps about killing other black people, praises drug dealers, and, in
one song, brags about drugging and raping a woman.

Looking back on what transpired, I do have to acknowledge that
I made a mistake—a couple of mistakes, actually. The first was for-
getting that Twitter isn't real life. It's troll farms and algorithms
designed to inflame. What feels like ten thousand people assaulting
you probably isn't. But like anyone who's been sucked into a social
media beatdown, I felt I couldn't log off without clarifying and coming back and doubling down again and again. I should have realized
sooner that the whole exercise was pointless. Ironically, there I was
all concerned about the effects social media was having on other
people, while failing to see the effects it was having on me.

When I dove headfirst into the online conversation about sexual
assault, I got plenty of backlash, but I was also swimming with the
tide of the prevailing sentiment. I was helping to amplify something

that was moving in the right direction. It's an entirely different experience to step out in front of a howling mob and say, "Hey, maybe we all need to stop and reflect on what we're doing and why we're doing it." Social media isn't built for any kind of nuanced, reasoned discussion. The mob is moving under its own power, and it won't stop until it drives itself over a cliff. Nothing you can say is going to be properly heard or understood.

I also have to acknowledge that my timing wasn't the best. When someone is injured or in pain, there's a lot of great advice you can give them about what they should do next, how they can recover and get back on their feet. But you can't hit them with that right away. Whether it's good advice or bad, they just don't want to hear it. You need to give them time to just sit and process their situation and be with their pain for a while.

I'm such a type A "You can do this! Let's tackle this! Go, go, go!" kind of person that I can forget that sometimes. In fact, I'd even forgotten it in that moment, in helping Rebecca recover from surgery. During those first months after the double mastectomy, in part because I was dealing with my own fears of losing her, I was going around being Mr. Positive. I was trying to force us to jump ahead to the place where everything would be okay again, and I was doing it to the point where, to her, it felt like I wasn't recognizing the pain she was in. It pissed her off. After she called me on it, I realized my mistake and I apologized.

Two weeks after George Floyd was killed, the nation was still in pain and in mourning. Everyone's emotions were still so raw. Regardless of how I felt or what I believed, what I said was not the right thing to say in the moment. I should have let tempers cool and wounds heal before I opened my mouth. I should have thought deliberately about the best way to articulate what I was trying to convey, rather than trying to fit it in under Twitter's character count. I should have

known that there was a better time, a better place, and a better me-
dium to say what I wanted to say.

Like maybe in a book.

Because I still believe the core of what I said is true. There is a
story about Frederick Douglass, the famous abolitionist, that I always keep in mind. Douglass was traveling the country, giving his
speeches, and the conductors of the railroad he was on wouldn't let
him sit in the first-class cabin with his white companions. They
made him sit in the back with the luggage. The white men traveling
with him were outraged and insulted on his behalf. They wanted to
lodge a protest, but Douglass refused, choosing to sit in the baggage
car instead. Douglass knew who he was, and therefore he could sit
anywhere and choose to be offended or not be offended. On that day,
getting to his speaking engagement on time was more important than
being offended, so he chose to do the former. "The soul that is within
me no man can degrade," Douglass said. "I am not the one that is
being degraded on account of this treatment but those who are in-
flicting it upon me."

Frederick Douglass understood power and agency in the same
way that Viktor Frankl understood power and agency. They come
from within. We can and should protest and call out injustice in the
world, but we cannot control or stamp out every injustice that exists.
What we can control, what we do have power over, is ourselves. We
can always choose what we say and how we respond. Martin Luther
King Jr. and Malcolm X and Fannie Lou Hamer and Shirley Chis-
holm understood that, too. Those men and women were able to endure everything from segregated rail cars to prison cells, because
nothing the world threw at them could dim the light they carried
inside themselves. That is true power.

The irony of the whole situation is that I failed to heed that lesson myself. When I sent my first tweet, I was trying to say, in essence, that all God's children needed to love one another, and that black people, in this heated moment, needed to listen to our better angels instead of succumbing to our worst selves. That's really all I wanted to say. But I didn't say that. I spoke too loud and too soon, and I let myself get dragged into a Twitter fight instead. I didn't wield the power of my voice as thoughtfully and judiciously as I should have. As for all the people who attacked my family and called me a clown and a race-traitor and a coon, I wonder if they have the humility to admit the same.

The Terry Crews–Black Supremacy social media maelstrom lasted about two and a half news cycles, which was two and a half more than it deserved. Fox News made hay out of it for a while. Don Lemon had me back on CNN, this time to drag me instead of celebrating me, and that wasn't great. And by the time it was done, still feeling defensive and misunderstood, I sent out my final thoughts on the matter:

> Are all white people bad? No. Are all black people
> good? No. Knowing this reality, I stand on my
> decision to unite with good people, no matter the
> race, creed or ideology. Given the number of threats
> against this decision, I also decide to die on this hill.

That's where I left it and, despite my missteps, that's where I still stand today. I believe that every black life should be not just protected but celebrated, but I want no part of any movement fueled by the impotent rage of victimhood. I want no part of any movement that doesn't begin with unity and reconciliation, because that is the only way for black lives in this country to truly flourish. The only future that allows our children to be whomever they choose to be is a future in which black America and white America reconcile and recognize that their fates are intertwined as one. I would argue that many if not most people agree with that premise, but the loudest voices in the room insist otherwise, and they're dragging us all in the wrong direction.

NEARLY FORTY YEARS AGO, after a childhood spent navigating between the two Michigans, I went to Interlochen Arts Camp, and I was given a gift. The judge who'd selected my paintings as the winners in the blind competition showed me how incredible it felt to be recognized simply as myself. I wasn't judged by the white preconceptions of who Terry Crews should be, and I wasn't judged by the black preconceptions of who Terry Crews should be. I was just Terry Crews. I spent decades in the NFL and in Hollywood trying to get to a place where I could feel that again, and it's taken me that long to understand that I don't need that judge or anyone else to give me that feeling. I have it every day now because I know that it comes from within.

Finding my way to that realization has taken a lifetime, and part of what has made it so difficult is being so ignorant of my past. On top of a lack of education about the history of race in school, my parents never told me their stories, because those stories were too painful to tell. Not knowing where I came from, I have always had that much harder a time understanding where I'm going. However, in the past year, even as I've been writing this book, I've managed to learn a few things that have blown my mind.

The first came through the opportunity to sit down with professor Henry Louis Gates Jr. for his PBS show *Finding Your Roots*. His researchers were able to trace parts of my family tree two hundred years into the past, which for a descendant of slavery is almost unheard of. "Terry," Professor Gates told me, "with African Americans, there are maybe two to three percent of the population where we can go back this far, just because the records don't exist."

What he found, on my mother's side, was the white family that owned my great-great-grandfather and his family: the Newsomes, in Sandersville, Georgia. He showed me the records, and it was like the Bible: "So-and-so begat so-and-so who begat so-and so." Only it's real people, your actual ancestors. I was in tears looking through them. It was so bittersweet, feeling not only the pain these people must have gone through but also the joy of discovering they existed.

In the earliest records, the black people didn't even have names. They were simply tracked like livestock: one black man, one wife, four boys. But Gates was able to deduce from the records that my great-great-grandparents had been separated at one point because the wife was sold away from the husband. Then, somehow, they worked it out that she could be sold back to the Newsome family so they could be together again.

Another amazing fact I learned was that five years after the Civil War, my family changed their last name from Newsome to Elbert, which I thought was brilliant. So many people kept their slave names moving forward. Some were so lost and overwhelmed in this new world of freedom that they turned right around and went back to the plantation and said, "Boss, I need a job," and moved back in as indentured servants. But the Elberts changed their name. We can only speculate as to why, but I like to think it was because they'd thrown off their slave mentality; they were determined to define themselves and live on their own terms and put the past behind them.

Interestingly, even as they changed their last name, they chose to name one of their children Kinchin, which was the name of Kinchin Newsome, the man who had owned them. Again, we can only speculate as to the reason, but as Gates explained it to me, even in the midst the brutality and evil of chattel slavery, there could still be relationships that were considered familial.

The second trove of information I discovered came from my dad's mother, Ermelle, whom we always called Seuk. She still lives in Edison, Georgia, and she turned ninety-four this year. I never really knew her because she was estranged from my father, but the fact that I'm her grandson and on TV every day gives her a lot of pride. She's made a few attempts to reach out and connect over the years. It was a little strange at first because we'd never had a relationship; I thought it was her wanting to talk to me because I got famous. Now I have a different perspective on it, which is that she's trying to make amends.

So I called Seuk on her ninety-fourth birthday, and I'm so glad I did. Because I finally got the story of my father's family. Seuk hadn't abandoned him, exactly. Seuk had had a hard life. She got pregnant by Edward Crews when she was sixteen. They were married two years later, but Edward's family treated her poorly because they were light skinned and she was dark skinned. On top of that, Edward Crews was a terrible husband and father. By the time my father was nine, Seuk sued Edward for abandonment of the children. He served nine months' hard labor at the Calhoun County Public Works Camp. When he got out he was arrested again, for the burglary of a liquor store, and sentenced to the chain gang. My father used to ride the bus to school, and he'd pass the chain gang inmates working the road, knowing that his father was out there on the chain. He was always nervous that other kids would tease him about it.

With her estranged husband in prison and no way to support herself, Seuk made the hard decision to send her children to live with Other Mama and Other Daddy, Katie and Claude Smart—not because she was abandoning them, as I'd been told, but because she had no choice. Four years after being released from prison, in 1963, Edward Crews died of an epileptic seizure at thirty-eight years old. My father was seventeen at the time. I was saddened to learn how difficult and painful his childhood had been. Still, it explained who he was and where he came from, and in that sense it felt good to hear. But the best part of that birthday call was that I finally got to learn about my great-grandfather Claude Smart.

Claude Smart was born in the late 1800s. He never had more than a third-grade education, but he learned to read and write, and he taught all the other black kids and even some of the grown-ups how to read and write, too. In fact, Claude Smart was so smart, and so capable, that once he grew up, the boss at the local lumber mill hired him on as a foreman, choosing him over several white guys for a job that, in those days, should have gone only to a white man. It caused such a firestorm in town that the white men who'd been passed over said that if Claude Smart showed up to work, they were going to kill him.

"We cried all day and all night," Seuk told me, "knowing there was a truck of white people on the way into town to kill my daddy. That night we were sitting in the house, hugging him and crying, and the next day he went to work knowing he was gonna die."

Claude Smart went to work that day, but he was clearly troubled, and the boss asked him what was wrong.

"Boss," he said, "they're going to kill me for taking this job."

"If they're going to kill you," the boss said, "they're going to have to kill me first."

The truck never showed up, and Claude Smart stayed at the mill and kept his job.

There are so many things I love about that story. First and

foremost is knowing that the story of my family isn't just a story of alcoholism and shame and abuse. It's also a story about nobility and strength and determination.

I also love that it's a more complicated story than most that get told about the history of this country. It's not a white-savior story, about some noble white man who saves the day while all the black folks just stand around. It's not a story of noble black people waging battle against some evil caricature of white people, either. It's about two men, my great-grandfather and his boss, who had to be willing to go against the grain. Both men had to have the courage to take a risk. Which is the only way anything in this world ever actually gets solved.

My whole childhood, Claude Smart was this legendary name that my dad used to invoke whenever things were going well or on those rare occasions he felt like he'd accomplished something good. Now I finally understood the greatness of what everyone was talking about when they talked about Claude Smart. And as we were wrapping up our call, Seuk said something that blew me away.

"You're like Claude Smart," she said. "He was so talented. We looked up to him like 'Oh my god, he could do anything,' and I see that in you."

Talking to Seuk and excavating my past with Professor Gates gave me a gift beyond measure. For the longest time, I looked back to my family's history and saw only dysfunction and despair. Now I'm able to look back and see strength and hope. Now I'm able to look back and finally understand the truth: I didn't come from my parents. I came through them. I can look into my past and see the bad and the good, and I can decide what part of the inheritance I want to carry forward with me.

The fact that my family changed their name and didn't see themselves as slaves anymore, that's mine. I'm taking that with me. The fact that my grandfather drank and stole and wound up on the chain gang, I choose to leave that behind. Because the fact is that the reason I exist is that my people never gave up. Even in the worst depths of slavery and oppression, they understood how to use the power that they had. Despite everything the world told them about who they were, they knew who they were. They stood tall and looked to the future, and saw me way off in the distance and thought, "Man . . . one day . . ."

And here I am.

EPILOGUE

I keep a picture in my office on my desk. It's a photo of me at six years old, my two front teeth missing. I keep it there so that I can always remember when I was good. I look at that picture, and I think, "Hey, man. There's nothing wrong with that kid. Absolutely not. He's a beautiful boy."

The kid in that picture doesn't know shame. He doesn't know racism or trauma or abuse. Since then I've done so many things that I regret, but the kid in that picture is innocent. He's not bad. Kids can't be bad. Children can cry, get mad, and throw their toys, but the truth is that, as children, we're inherently good, and I use the goodness of my childhood self as a compass. That smiling, gap-toothed kid in the picture, that's who I was before life happened to me, and while I'll never be that innocent again, the photo is a reminder that I can be that good again if I try.

And I do try. It's taken me ten years of nonstop working on

myself, but I've finally come to a better place. I don't use my muscles to beat people up anymore. I use them to build things. I've learned to sit and be sad, to acknowledge my weakness and vulnerability. I practice empathy every day, not just with my wife and kids and co-workers, but even with the guy who cuts me off in traffic. Even that guy is not an object I need to control. He's a person in a hurry I need to try to understand, and the more I understand and empathize with him, the better I feel, because I don't get angry.

When I do get angry, I've learned to manage it. I don't fly off the handle anymore. I don't snap. I've literally rewired my neural pathways to work differently. I feel the anger coming on, I identify the source of it, and I ask myself, "Why am I letting this make me angry? Oh, I'm getting angry because I have an unrealistic expectation of how this other person should be acting. I need to let that go." Or, "I thought this person was antagonizing me, but really it's a miscommunication. I need to let that go." And I do.

Most important, I work every day to be a better husband and a better father. My marriage has never been in a better place. I've had a harder time with my older daughters, the ones who lived through all those years of my toxic behavior. I ask for and work for their forgiveness every day. It hasn't been easy, but we're making progress. My son, being the youngest, was spared the worst, and our relationship is a revelation to me. He wants to learn from everything that I do, and I encourage him in everything he does—and we *talk*. He knows he can always ask me anything. It's amazing. My relationship with him is the exact opposite of my relationship with my own parents.

As for my parents, that has been the steepest road of all. Where my father and I simply didn't speak for ten years after the Christmas from Hell, Trish and I always stayed in touch. She was proud of me for making it in Hollywood. She would brag about me all the time.

One of the highlights of actually succeeding out here was seeing her being happy that I was doing it. By that point in her life, my mother wasn't letting religion control her as much, which was wonderful to see. She'd become more free in every respect. She would go to the movies and listen to secular music and even wear blue jeans.

I'd do my best to keep an eye on things with her and Big Terry. She would never tell me anything, but I knew their health and their financial situation wasn't good. At one point she moved out. "I'm living with some friends now," she told me, when really she was at a shelter for battered women. She just wouldn't admit it. Around that time, Rebecca and I were finally getting on our feet, and I begged her to come out and live with us, but Trish wouldn't hear of it. "No, no, I'm fine," she said. "I love Michigan. I love my friends. I've got Faith Tech. I've got all my stuff here. Why would I be out there with you?" Two years later she was back living with Big Terry again.

It was the same thing when she got sick. She came for a visit and I noticed a swelling in her neck. She went back to Flint and was diagnosed with non-Hodgkin's lymphoma and had to start aggressive chemotherapy. I asked her to please come out and live with us, where I could take her to see some better doctors, and again she said no. Luckily, her treatment worked and the cancer went into remission.

Then, a year after I got out of rehab in Arizona, while trying to take inventory of my past, rebuild my marriage, and put my life back together, I reached out to my mom. I was conscious of the fact that I might not have much time left with her. I wanted us to set things right before she was gone. So I called her and I brought up the subject of my childhood abuse, all the hitting and the slapping and particularly the time she'd forced me to expose myself to show her if I'd gone through puberty. She immediately recoiled at the mention of it. "I didn't do anything like that," she said.

"Yes, you did."

"No, I would have remembered something like that."

"Ma, you did it," I said, "And it was severely disturbing."

She got real angry and blew up at me and ended the phone call. A month later, I sat down and wrote her a letter.

Hi Ma,

I hope this letter finds you well. I've been here in Bulgaria filming Expendables 2 for over a month and I've had a lot of time to think. Mostly about life and my relationships. I am sad about how our last conversation ended, but I'm also happy that some things were put out in the open. I know where you are and you know how I feel about things. That's always a good thing. I'm forever grateful for the love and sacrifices you made in raising me. You kept me on the straight and narrow, and I always tell people my sense of humor comes from you. The laughs we've shared are precious and my fondest memories as a child is of trying to make you laugh.

I want to rebuild my relationship with you from the ground up. I believe sometimes things have to be dismantled, examined, cleaned then put back together so they work correctly. I understand if you don't want to—but if you could allow me to shoot you these notes from time to time, I would be grateful. I want you in my life. Plain and simple. I apologize for any hurt I have caused you and I forgive you for any of the same. I just had to finally acknowledge some things that happened that I've always struggled with in order to move past them. I'm done. And if there's anything more on your side that you'd like to share with me I am anxious to hear it. I humbly ask you to please understand that I was not trying to hurt you.

I love you, I care for you and I believe things can be repaired,
and I will continue to do so.

> *Thank you for listening,*
> *Your son*

She wrote back:

Of course without reservations you can contact me as
many times as you want. I too have had time to think about
our conversation. . . . I would hope we can be angry at each
other without unforgiveness keeping us from having a loving
relationship. I am truly sorry for any hurt I have caused you
in the past and I would love for us to have an honest and
sincere relationship. You are my son and I love you very much.
Anything you want to talk to me about you can but let's do it
in a civil manner and agree to disagree and still love each
other. I have reached the age where there are many regrets
in my life but there are three things I do not regret . . .
Marcelle, Lil Terry and Michaell . . . you three are my greatest
accomplishments and I want my babies to be happy and live
lives of fullness and productivity. . . . I have not always been
the greatest mother but one thing I can say . . . is that I tried to
do my best and I will admit my wrongs and try to do better in
the future. . . . I am now 62 and still growing and changing. . . .
I know you were not trying to hurt me and I wasn't hurt to the
point where I couldn't understand YOUR pain. . . . Life is too
short to be unforgiving but I wanted to let you have your space
if that is what you wanted. . . . All things are possible with
Jesus Christ and I believe you and I can have a relationship

if we are willing to work at it and I am more than willing
to do so.

Love,

Trish

After that, Trish and I both began to heal. It felt incredible, and as difficult as confronting the past was, I'm so glad I chose to do it, because soon her cancer was back. That same year she started chemo again and fought for four more years.

In the end, it wasn't the cancer that took her. One day she woke up feeling sick, and Big Terry took her to the hospital, where she sat around for days, untreated and undiagnosed. Then a nurse took note of the fact that this poor black woman was "Terry Crews's mother." Now the hospital cared. They ran more tests and identified an infection that had been coursing through her body all the days she'd been lying in bed untreated. They airlifted her to Henry Ford Hospital in Detroit, but by then, it was too late. The infection had spread to her brain. I got to speak to her on her deathbed, but she was barely coherent by that point.

She died two days before Thanksgiving. It was a sunny Los Angeles day when I got the news. I was standing in the kitchen, and I looked outside and all I could see were bright billowing clouds. It felt like she was part of them. I didn't cry. What I felt was a tremendous sense of peace, because I'd had the chance to share all my thoughts and feelings with her before she passed, and that meant everything in the world.

For a long time, I hoped my father and I would find our way back to a similar place. When I came out of therapy, I knew he'd stopped drinking again, and I wanted to open the door for a reconciliation between us. Before I called him, however, I knew I had to think of one great thing that he did for me in order to be thankful and acknowledge who he was in my life. To be honest, I couldn't think of much. But at the end of the day he is my father, and the simple fact is that without him and whatever happened in his life that led him to my mother, I wouldn't exist. From that perspective, I owe him everything. So I called him up and said, "Big Terry, I want to thank you for having me, because I wouldn't be here without you, and that's enough to just tell you thank you."

That man cried like I had never heard him cry before. Then he apologized for everything he'd ever done. "I'm so sorry," he said. "I was so mean to you guys and your mom, and I'm so sorry."

On my next trip back to Flint, I took him out to breakfast and we talked some things out that we hadn't talked about in a long time. It wasn't acrimonious at all. It was healing. "This is what it's all about," I thought, "acknowledging the past and learning from it, and then leaving it behind to move on with our lives."

After breakfast, we were out in the parking lot, and I went to hug Big Terry. Then, the moment my arms locked around him, I couldn't let him go. I hugged him like I hugged when I was four years old, really squeezing him tight. For a minute, I felt him tense up. Then he relaxed into it and I kept on holding him and he let me. I never could have imagined his letting me hug him like that before. I'd been trapped in my stunted view of manliness, I wouldn't have been able to do it, either.

I thought we were on a new path. Then, around the time my mother died, he started drinking again, and it all fell apart. He started calling me up out of nowhere, drunk and belligerent, saying things like "You ain't shit." Usually it was about how I wouldn't give him any money, which I wouldn't. Then, after the Adam Venit thing, it became all about that. "You're pathetic. You're not a man. You're an embarrassment to the family."

The last straw came when he called me up and berated me ten

minutes before I was about to go onstage and host an episode of *America's Got Talent: The Champions.* When I got onstage, it was impossible to perform with his voice ringing in my head. I tried to shake it off, but I couldn't. He's my father. There I was on TV entertaining millions of people, and in my head I felt like a scared and worthless seven-year-old boy.

The next afternoon I called him back and said, "Okay, Big Terry. You want money, so I'm just curious: How much would it cost me for you to never call me again?"

He didn't miss a beat. "Ten thousand dollars," he said.

It knocked the wind out of me.

"Huh?"

Because that was not the answer I was expecting. I'd been expecting to him to say, "You're my son. I love you. There's no amount of money that could ever stop me from talking to you." Nope. Not even close. Ten grand. He even had the figure right off the top of his head. That was brutal. I never paid him the money; I always wanted to keep the door open for us to start talking again. But I also knew I had to step back and insulate myself from the abuse. I changed my phone number, and we didn't talk for three years, which hurt like hell.

Just recently—two weeks ago as I'm writing this—he reached back out to try to make amends. He admitted he'd fallen off the wagon when my mother died, which he'd lied about for years. I told him I'd buy him a truck so he could get back to making some money doing some handyman jobs around town.

It's a start.

ACKNOWLEDGMENTS

I want to thank my wife, Rebecca; my kids, Naomi, Azriel, Tera, Wynfrey, Isaiah; and my granddaughter, Miley; my uncle Sonny Crews, for all the valuable information; my manager, Troy Zien; my agents at UTA, Albert Lee, Jo Yao, Sam Stone, Scott Schachter, Chris Hart, Andrew Lear, Matt Rice, and Spencer Goldstein; my attorney, David Krintzman; Lifeline Business Managers, Humble Lukanga, Brandon Burnett, and Garrett Ray; Nana Boateng, Dakota Xentaras, and Hannah Haas; my publicist, Haley Hileman; Jim and Marguerite Reeve; Ken and Janice Harvey; Dr. Henry Louis Gates Jr., Bear Grylls, Adam Grant, and Amanda Nguyen.

I want to especially thank Leah Trouwborst, Trish Daly, Tanner Colby, and everyone at Portfolio and Penguin Random House for this amazing opportunity to tell my story.